Treating the Patient with a Traumatic Past

Treating the Patient with a Traumatic Past

A Guide for Clinicians

Patricia E. Moyer
Assistant Professor of Medicine, Harvard Medical School Core Internal Medicine Faculty
Mt. Auburn Hospital, Cambridge, MA

OXFORD
UNIVERSITY PRESS

OXFORD
UNIVERSITY PRESS

Oxford University Press is a department of the University of Oxford. It furthers the University's objective of excellence in research, scholarship, and education by publishing worldwide. Oxford is a registered trade mark of Oxford University Press in the UK and in certain other countries.

Published in the United States of America by Oxford University Press
546 Fifth Avenue, New York, NY 10036, United States of America

Library of Congress Cataloging-in-Publication Data
Names: Moyer, Patricia (Patricia E.) author
Title: Treating the patient with a traumatic past : a guide for clinicians / Patricia E. Moyer.
Description: New York, NY : Oxford University Press, 2026. |
Includes bibliographical references and index.
Identifiers: LCCN 2026013176 (print) | LCCN 2026013177 (ebook) |
ISBN 9780190250751 pb | ISBN 9780190250768 | ISBN 9780190250775 epub |
ISBN 9780190250782
Subjects: LCSH: Patient-centered health care | Trauma-informed care |
Physicians (General practice)—Vocational guidance | Adult child abuse
victims—Medical care | Psychic trauma—Treatment
Classification: LCC R727.38 .M69 2026 (print) | LCC R727.38 (ebook)
LC record available at https://lccn.loc.gov/2026013176
LC ebook record available at https://lccn.loc.gov/2026013177

DOI: 10.1093/med/9780190250751.001.0001

Printed by Integrated Books International, United States of America

The manufacturer's authorized representative in the EU for product safety is Oxford University Press España S.A. of Parque Empresarial San Fernando de Henares, Avenida de Castilla, 2 – 28830 Madrid (www.oup.es/en or product.safety@oup.com). OUP España S.A. also acts as importer into Spain of products made by the manufacturer.

MIX
Paper
FSC FSC® C183721

Contents

Preface vii
Acknowledgments xi

1. The Intersection of Violence and General Medicine 1
2. Disclosure 14
3. Post-Traumatic Stress Disorder 30
4. Dissociation 63
5. Power and Control 85
6. Self-Harm 106
7. Trauma and the Body 135
8. The Doctor–Patient Relationship 161
9. Abuse, Violence, and Medical Care: Toward a Trauma-Informed System 175
10. The End 198

Index 211

Preface

This book has been written over the course of many years. During that time much has changed in the practice of medicine. The computer has become a staple in the exam room. Governments have raised and enforced standards of what constitutes "quality" medical care. Dashboards, templates, and guidelines greet practitioners at every turn, hoping to "streamline" care and promote its value to all.

If we can keep our focus, one thing has not changed. That one thing is the phenomenon of sitting in a private spot with a human being hoping for better health, and engaging with them in a relationship toward that goal. Keeping this at the heart of what we do is one of the sources of joy in the practice of medicine.

My journey began back in medical school in New York, at the Albert Einstein College of Medicine in the Bronx. We students were set loose with plenty of time, though as yet little experience, with very sick people and allowed to accompany them during their illnesses, to learn from what happened to them and us. I was fortunate back then to have an array of wise mentors, and no shortage of patients from whom to learn. Later, during residency at what is now the Cambridge Health Alliance, I had the chance to try to emulate a number of excellent caregivers, who were not afraid to bring their real selves into the consulting room. Still further on, I became acquainted with "patient-centered interviewing." This seemed to involve a sort of readiness to wander where patients' inflected language might lead, while paradoxically keeping an orderly diagnostic or therapeutic path alive in the mind. Pretty soon, I began hearing things that had never been in my medical textbooks or lectures.

The spectrum of disease, diagnosis, and therapeutics is broad and endlessly fascinating. (This is one reason why a group of clinicians can so easily descend into "shop talk.") I have found nothing as interesting, however, as exploring, with a patient's consent, what they really mean by a stray word, a surprise emotion, or an obscure reference. Quickly, we can get "off topic" and, at the same time, on to the real chase. Learning how to do this within the constraints of time and fairness to oneself, and to all of one's patients, is doable but takes time.

The increasing presence and importance of "physician extenders"—physician assistants, nurse practitioners, midwives—in the primary care workforce, and the increasing power and voice of nursing professionals, has extended the gamut of who may be a primary professional sitting with a patient. I've been trained as a physician, and from that experience often refer in this book to caregivers as doctors. However, I've worked shoulder to shoulder with excellent non-doctor clinicians for several decades. Whether I use the word doctor, clinician, professional, or caregiver, I mean to imply any of these medical professionals working in an ongoing primary relationship with a patient. My hope is to reach into the worlds that we all inhabit. There are distinctions, but there are many similarities when it comes to matters discussed here.

Another source of "blur" while writing has occurred in the course of identifying provider gender. The reader may notice that I move back and forth with personal pronouns when discussing various hypothetical situations between providers and patients. Sometimes, patients will select a provider of one gender or another for their own comfort. Often, however, we providers are thrown together with patients somewhat randomly—with genders the same as or different from our own. Some patients and providers prefer an identity not limited by gender identification. I move in this volume between "he" and "she" in referring to professionals, but acknowledge that some are "they." The book was largely written during a time when the term *they* was not in use. Chiefly, I want to acknowledge that victims and perpetrators of childhood trauma can be male, female, or neither, and that providers can be these as well. Importantly, however, healers must call on personal traits traditionally ascribed to male and female genders in order to be effective with survivors of childhood trauma. They may need to learn to be both encouraging, receptive, and good listeners, and decisive, active, outspoken, or irreverent as the situation demands.

Mostly, I did not change the gender of those serving as my named patient examples. I disguised a great deal in presenting their situations in order to protect their identity. But I felt it was important for my readers to understand that trauma, including sexual and military trauma, can happen to a young person of any gender and is common to all.

All the patients appearing in this volume represent something about the people I have cared for over 40 years. Everyone's identity has been disguised. Those patients (the majority) with whom I have had an ongoing relationship have read and had input into their stories, how they were presented, and have consented to and encouraged me to use our work together to educate the medical profession. Some patients have passed away. A few patients have moved on, often many years ago, and I have not been able to locate them. In this case

I constructed composite patients and composite problems but attempted to retain what was true to my own actions and reactions, successes and failures.

In reviewing their chapters, forming revisions, and giving consent, a number of patients have courageously come forward to you, the reader, with stories of their past that are still affecting their lives and their health today. These are not easy, happy times to revisit. The losses and damage are real. Some of my patients were angry, frightened, shaken, or grief-stricken as they reviewed what has happened to them and thought about how it still impacts them. We needed time together to work through all of this. Ultimately, we came to share what these patients felt really mattered about the impact of prior trauma on health. It is with their sacrifices in mind that this book is offered to you.

Acknowledgments

Writing is a deeply personal venture that entices the author into hours of solitude. At the same time, along the way, interactions with many people encourage one deeply. My work on this book has rested firmly, all along, on such nurturers.

Treatment had its genesis in two relationships and experiences. The first was parenting my then-adolescent son—who learns best by doing, trial, and error—while he suffered his way through an academic, left-brain high school education. What, he asked me one night at dinner, had I done with *my* fine and expensive education that made it at all worthwhile? I was practicing medicine steadily and reliably, but had I risen out of myself to create anything in my own voice, anything that changed the world? This uncannily perceptive teenage complaint formed the nub of a lasting disturbance.

A second experience was more grueling. A beloved and cherished member of my wider religious community, who spent a great deal of time and energy working with the group's young people, was felt by some to have transgressed boundaries of touch and intimacy with some of the children. Opinions on his activity were strong and deeply divided. As part of a group tasked with finding a way forward, I found myself in relation with this individual with gifts, charisma, and, it seemed to me, an overweening self-confidence which brooked no opposition. Interacting with him and his many supporters was an education in subtlety, boundaries, and the muscular powers which drive people to shape their world and the people they meet. I realized how important the lines are that must be drawn; how relentless are the forces that would cross those lines, and how much energy is needed to contain those forces—energy that I had to reach deeply into myself to muster.

I thank the faithful members of my support committee from Fresh Pond Meeting of the Religious Society of Friends (Quakers), Karin Downs, William How (deceased), Lawrence Kessenich, and Lynn Hart Taber. Their belief in my work with the above-named individual, and subsequently in this book and in my ability to write it, helped keep me soldiering on, especially when my doubts loomed large. Their collective skills and experience in advocating for the health of women and children, overseeing the state's concern for children in potentially abusive families, writing well, and in the profession of nursing, with attention to children and families, made for many rich evenings together over the years. The understandings we developed concerning boundary violators, victims, and our social fabric were invaluable to me.

I am indebted to the Society of Friends itself for educating us all in the concept of clearness and support committees, formed to help people navigate the leadings of the Spirit in living on earth.

The Rabkin Fellowship in Medical Education, begun at Mt. Auburn Hospital in Cambridge, Massachusetts, and shepherded by Drs. Charles Hatem and Beth Lown, provided me with a space for weekly reflection and inquiry about teaching, learning, and initiative, over the course of one year. The work I began during that year has evolved into this volume. This book might not have happened if Dr. Ayse Atasoylu had not been a fellow with me during that year, listened to one of my stories, and concluded, with piercing eye contact, that I needed to write this book. Her remark went into my soul and has not left me since. Dr. Matthew Carmody, another member of the fellowship, cleared and maintained a listening space at an important time, a model for some of what this book envisions.

More recently, I've been fortunate enough to have joined the Z Street writers, a group of seven women who critique and encourage each other's poetry, in regular meetings, to improve their craft. Their acceptance, curiosity, deep support, and intelligent, attentive feedback have helped me think about words and their meaning.

I owe an enormous debt of gratitude to Dr. Barbara Pizer, who encouraged this work and regularly reminded me of its importance.

My husband, Bruce Neumann, has made most of our hot meals over the last few years and learned to travel softly by the door of my study when I'm riveted to the screen. He has endured many an hour of silence which the revisions of this work seemed to need. His has been a sensitive support.

Finally, I thank my patients, who have trusted me with themselves, their health, and their stories. I work to deserve this trust. I hope that we can all gain from their sharing.

1

The Intersection of Violence and General Medicine

Introduction

About 30 years ago, Dr. James Gilligan published a little volume entitled *Violence* (1), in which he discussed the nature and treatment of men imprisoned for acts of major crimes against others. Writing from his 10-year experience as psychiatric treatment director at Bridgewater State Hospital in Massachusetts, he explored the "pathology," the "germ theory," and the "epidemiology" of violence. He describes, using stark yet compassionate examples, the inner "deadness" of the man who has harmed others—a death that happened before he became a criminal, at the hands of human beings who were supposed to nurture him. He also postulates that the roots of violent behavior lie not in this lack of feeling but in the feeling beneath that, of intense personal shame. Violence, Gilligan says, is done to avenge shame, to avoid the feeling of shame, to expiate shame, to erase shame—to appear to self and others as fully "a man"—a cultural ideal not compatible with shame.

For most of his patients, shame grew from their early days at the hands of their family, their lack of family, their school system, our social institutions, and our culture. One chapter is entitled, "The Deadliest Form of Violence is Poverty."

Gilligan does not excuse his patients' behaviors in any way. He gives unflinching accounts of their violent acts to help us understand who they really are. He does not excuse himself, either. Late in the book, he reflects on what his role in the violent death of one of his patients, in the hospital, might have been. He dedicates his book "to all the victims of violence: past, present, and future." I highly recommend it.

The book which you hold in your hands also proposes to look at these issues of violence and its treatment, but from the point of view of the recipients of violence—in particular, those who were youth when it happened to them. Like the Bridgewater residents, these victims also suffer deep shame, among other powerful emotions. Instead of criminal behavior, though, their life journeys involve physical and psychic syndromes, and the onset of disease, which then lead them to doctors' offices. While the "criminally insane" are relatively few, these people are many in number. Strikingly, what has happened to them has also occurred within families, by neighbors, and within institutions such as churches, clinics, the military, camps, and schools, all of which exist to guard, educate, and lead children into healthy adulthood.

While the poor, minorities, and males are greatly over-represented in prisons, the victims of violence which this book examines may be of any class, race, or gender. Many are women. Most of them, unlike Gilligan's patients, are not easily identifiable. Because the outcomes of trauma for these people are so heterogeneous, and so numerous, it's impossible to make a single description which fits all. Yet, I believe, their past experiences with violence have set them on a trajectory of suffering that can best be understood and remediated by getting to its roots. Because health care institutions and practitioners exist to treat suffering, we practitioners need to better understand the basis, in violence, of these patients' symptoms. In order to properly care for adults who have been traumatized as children—in order, really, to care for anyone who has experienced trauma (including the traumas of illness, loss, and death)—medical clinicians need an education and an understanding of the positive roles they themselves may play.

I have written this book while reflecting on my own numerous experiences in general medicine, caring for a wide variety and number of patients whose histories encompass a story of childhood trauma. Sometimes such stories were remembered by patients; sometimes they were recognized as such, and many times they were not—certainly not early in our relationship. General medicine and primary care offer its practitioners the gift of knowing people through time. My patients and I have had symptom variety, memory, and trust-building as aids in understanding their issues. Their paths have shed light on my own, as well.

Because I am a female doctor, many women have come to me with problems which originated in childhood sexual trauma. There seems to be a great deal of that in American society. However, not infrequently, I and others discover histories of sexual trauma of boys, physical trauma to both sexes, boundary violations, men and women soldiers burdened with wartime violence, and legacies of emotional abuse. Often, there are sequential stories of abuse, or combinations which occur simultaneously or over time.

How do we know what we are seeing? A medical relationship might begin with a doctor, a person seeking care, and a problem needing remedy—or perhaps just the desire for a trustworthy, confidential relationship. At the outset, more is on everyone's mind than is spoken. The patient: get this problem solved, I am worried, how is this doctor handling my problem, how many of the rules can I live with, do I like him/her? The doctor: can I get this done in a timely fashion? Is this something I know how to deal with? Why this problem, now? Do I like this person? Is there another story? What do I do with the fleeting thoughts in my head? Why did s/he pick me? Does it bear on anything?

Most of these thoughts and feelings are not uttered. Some are hardly consciously experienced. Some are communicated; many are not. Occasionally our written narrative catches some of them or serves as a proxy for recalling them later.

There is not much time or space in our first meetings for asking the bigger questions, nor, usually, is there a need. Reviewing my cases longitudinally has taught me something, however. Clues about a patient's bigger story (our concern here being childhood trauma) are often present right away. They are present in the problems brought to the clinician, in the way in which the person handles herself, and in the ways in which the relationship—doctor/patient—unfolds.

Symptoms and Clues

What is confusing and confounding about practicing medicine is that many things can mean many things. Consider this list, written by the American College of Obstetrics and Gynecology (ACOG), meant to inform obstetricians and gynecologists of possible presentations of prior sexual abuse:

Common Symptoms in Adult Survivors of Childhood Sexual Abuse

Physical Presentations
- Chronic pelvic pain
- Gastrointestinal symptoms/distress
- Musculoskeletal complaints
- Obesity, eating disorders
- Insomnia, sleep disorders
- Pseudocyesis
- Sexual dysfunction
- Asthma, respiratory ailments
- Addiction
- Chronic headache
- Chronic back pain

Psychologic and Behavioral Presentations
- Depression and anxiety
- Post-traumatic stress disorder symptoms
- Dissociative states
- Repeated self-injury
- Suicide attempts
- Lying, stealing, truancy, running away
- Poor contraceptive practices
- Compulsive sexual behaviors
- Sexual dysfunction
- Somatizing disorders
- Eating disorders
- Poor adherence to medical recommendations
- Intolerance of or constant search for intimacy
- Expectation of early death (2).

In my own experience, this "laundry list" is valid. Such symptoms and states *are* common among adult survivors. But could not this list represent one's entire waiting area on any given day? Surely not *everyone* out there is a survivor of child sexual abuse. Are they?

I suspect the purpose of the list, and the article in which it is embedded, was to awaken clinicians and to educate them about the existence of childhood sexual abuse and its manifestations in adult survivors. As such, it was extremely valuable. What all of us may need, however, is a sense of where to go next. Given that many of these common complaints and states COULD represent prior abuse, and that many of the people who see us every day about them might therefore have been abused, what do we do? I hope to provide some answers in this chapter and in this book.

For now, let's look at a case which embodies such ambiguity. It has no answers, just questions, and I suspect it will feel familiar to many of you.

Oliver

Many years ago, Oliver saw one of my associates for his first visit to our practice. He was in the middle of middle-age. He was concerned about a pain in his right thumb, though it was not currently bothering him. Might it be work-related? He had seasonal allergies. When asked for past medical history, he did not wish to discuss it, as he felt healthy. My colleague told him to come back if his hand hurt again.

He came in next several months later to see me with a minor rash, which looked inflamed. He was a slight, middle-aged man. He looked young for his age, mildly depressed, and was dressed in such a way that he did not call attention to himself. He and I could not understand the cause of the rash.

Two months later he saw me because of a three- to four-year history of a change in bowel function. He had had intermittent constipation, a change in stool appearance and texture, and had spasms of rectal pain, lasting up to two or three minutes at a time. He allowed me to examine his abdomen and rectum. There were no unusual findings. I recommended a barium enema and a flexible sigmoidoscopy, and some Metamucil, suspecting Oliver might have irritable bowel syndrome, at least. I wondered about "something else" with his rectum—it puzzled me, though I didn't say how. He was to return after the tests. Six weeks later, he called me while he was on a holiday. He didn't want to have the tests; he felt anxious, and said he didn't want anyone seeing him in a johnny. The Metamucil was helping. I wondered why he was calling at this odd time about something he'd clearly been brooding about for months. I felt a little more "invited" into his space. He canceled the tests, despite a discussion of risks and benefits. He promised to reschedule them.

He came in a few times because of low back pain, which he attributed to his job. He did not want to tell me where he worked or what he did, declaring this "irrelevant," but did say that he was in front of a computer a lot. He asked again about the barium x-rays, did not want them scheduled, and wanted to know what personal information I was writing in his chart. I told him I had almost no personal information to enter.

At the end of that year, however, he did come in for his first physical exam. He came into my office for the interview portion, my custom at the time for a first long visit. He then became quite upset. I had patient charts and x-rays in the room (this was well before the time of electronic records.) What kind of guarantees, he asked, could I give him about his private information? Desk charts and piles had sometimes occasioned jokes or sympathy from patients about my workload. No one had ever confronted me like this. I was floored. I felt irresponsible and ashamed, guilty as charged, and gave Oliver the option of skipping his exam or of seeing another doctor. I felt in the moment that my way of working must have violated some basic professional code of conduct, in his mind at least.

It only occurred to me afterwards that this interchange might be symptomatic of **his** issues with safety, hiding, and being known. Shame was alive in the room, and I had assumed it was all mine. Now things seemed even more confusing. Whose problem was I treating?

Oliver did not seem to connect the chart piles with having a physical. He still wanted it and went through it in a matter-of-fact way. Notably, his history was scant and his exam unremarkable.

A couple of months later, while we were in an exam room together for a minor complaint, Oliver told me how he had felt about talking in my office. He had thought being ushered in was going to result in an invitation to leave the practice! This also shocked me. After reacting with anxiety to chart piles I had, and feeling I should have hidden them more completely, he was now revealing his own vulnerability—having done nothing at all wrong or offensive. Some people have told me after coming into my office that they expect some special interchange; or they tell me (year after year) that I have a new view from the window. But I could think of nothing which would have given Oliver the idea that I would dismiss him. Again, it did not occur to me that perhaps **he** would rather have not been there to experience the intimacy of a medical history and physical.

These incidents have haunted me through the years, perhaps because they were so informative. They taught me. Important feelings, memories, structures can be evoked in the encounter, and the clinician's awareness of them—in self or other—are valuable clues. Doctor and patient together must sort out their source, over time, with the doctor's self-knowledge and experience as an anchor. Also, I see now, Oliver's willingness to be vulnerable came after he stirred up (his? my?) shame. Finally, this happened both times so quickly, both of us so naïve, that there was no way I could have understood all of it at the time.

Oliver, at his first full exam, would not tell me where he was born or brought up, or where he was living or working now. He said he was estranged from his family, except for a cousin. We went through a conventional review of systems but seem not to have discussed much about whether he was currently sexually active, or with whom. He had been "thinking about it," he said.

He made poor eye contact. His exam was otherwise normal. I referred him for a colonoscopy, due to the increasing awareness of colonoscopy as the preferred screening modality for colon cancer. He was now well over 50. Sometime later he called to tell me he would not go through with it. He had found out that he had to get a ride home and told me that he had no one in his life whom he could ask for a ride. I suggested he just go meet the gastroenterologist, and left it at that.

Over the next few years, Oliver showed up for several physicals. At one, he had quit taking Metamucil, as it was "too expensive." At several, he refused a genital and rectal exam. He would not discuss whether or not he was sexually active. He appeared depressed, but considered questions about his feelings intrusive. At his most recent visit, he told me without much ado where he was working and how he felt about it. He mentioned a visit with his cousin. He continued to refuse genital and rectal exams, but seemed a bit more relaxed in my company. He never had the colonoscopy.

Reflections

What can we learn from Oliver's case? Is this a case of prior abuse, sexual or otherwise? I can only suspect so. I really have no idea. His presence and our interactions raised the questions of trust, secrecy, sharing, family distance, neglect, harm, and professionalism. His symptoms and scant history referred my thinking to his genitals and his lower GI tract. What else has happened to them? Or to what body experience might they refer? He manifests several items from the ACOG list (written about women, not men): "GI symptoms and distress, (possible) sexual dysfunction (we don't really know), dissociative states, and poor adherence to medical recommendations." Are all of these enough to broach the topic of prior abuse with Oliver?

More questions arise. How should I have handled his first arrival for a complete exam? I felt it was an attack—on me, my office, my professional self. Because I was so flustered, I immediately reminded him he could leave, that this was his choice. How could I, instead, have used his distress as an opening? Then the turn of the tables—he had "thought" that my invitation to a bit greater intimacy heralded my asking **him** to leave. How much of that could I have explored? Meanwhile, I was too taken aback to think on my feet, either time. Rather than reflect his behavior back to him, I offered him a choice—stay or leave. I was angry, unsettled, frightened. Underneath, I worried about my possibly too-casual approach to charts, and not Oliver's extreme concerns about remaining anonymous—that didn't even occur to me.

My experience is that specific recommendations for colonoscopy in particular, with every good intention and reason, often fall flat for people who have endured child abuse, especially sexual abuse. This is a group for whom seeing Katie Couric's colon on TV is just not enough. When Oliver is confronted with needing one, he suddenly has no friends, no acquaintances—no one he can "burden" with his relatively minor needs. At the prospect of one, he appears to feel truly alone in the world. That might be very telling.

I chose never to bring up the subject of abuse to Oliver. For one thing, our license to explore together—the ownership of which must always belong to him—is very limited. He hasn't presented many opportunities to go beyond. In fact, he spends quite a bit of time shutting the doors on my open-ended questions. My job seems to be to honor those limits. His question to me is, mainly, will you take care of me even if I give you very little to work with? Eventually, after a number of years and without fanfare or goodbye, he left the practice. I don't know why.

I was never sure of my suspicions. Though Oliver exhibits symptoms on the ACOG list, we have discussed how non-specific they are and how multiple their possible meanings and relationships. Could these be these true for men, too? I feel too unclear about the possibility, overly intrusive if I ask, and as if the major issues here are trust, reliability, and acceptance. Despite his concerns, and my imperfect handling of them, he returned, on his own schedule, many times over the period of a decade or so. He has continued to hold my recommendations in mind and has managed to share a little more with me about himself. So that is where we had to leave it.

Professional Response to Childhood Trauma

I spoke earlier about preparing to be better doctors for the Olivers of the world. We might start by educating ourselves about violence in our society. We can think about its presence, our strangely elusive understanding of its presence, its definitions, and its prevalence.

In its 2002 report, *Confronting Chronic Neglect* (3), the Institute of Medicine detailed the state of violence education among health care professionals in the United States. They decried the lack of content and time devoted to family violence education across the board—from professional schools, to residency, and to continuing education. Missing, too, they said, were studies detailing what should be learned and by whom; and studies of what works.

Surgeons learn early and continuously how to repair the physical wounds of accidents, assault, and war. When, as a profession, can we learn to listen for, identify, witness, and promote healing from those and other traumas which people endure? As a people, we first must admit not only that such things happen but that they are intolerable. This is not just the task of professional schools. It seems to be very difficult for us all to admit, or to contemplate, or to endure our feelings about such things as fathers sexually stimulating their daughters and "enjoying" it, about abduction of children on the way home from school, about camp counselors eroticizing their jobs with our offspring, or about young women military recruits being sexually assaulted by their peers and ignored by their superiors.

We can perhaps examine how we each feel, thinking about that last sentence, as a clue to some of the difficulties our society faces as a whole. We would rather that such events never, ever happened. We would hope that such a thing could never happen to our children, at least. We would like to live with the construct that we can arrange our family's and friends' lives so that we never need worry about violence to our children. We can hope that if we follow the advice of experts and educators, and teach our children well what to do, that they will be protected. If such a catastrophe does happen to someone in our community, it might be best if we could "explain" it in such a way that it would make it seem unlikely ever to happen to us. We can assign blame to the victim ("She knew better than to be walking there alone") or to her parents ("They don't spend enough time with their kids").

Or perhaps we feel that such criminal activity, while not tolerable, is private and within the confines of the home. We are not far from the days when we felt that "a man's home is his castle" and by deduction, who was the king? It seemed worse to intrude on the privacy of the home, and its doings, than to protect the rights of the children and the women or other men who lived there.

There might be a part of us that feels that the whole notion of victimization is unhealthy—something that, in assuming or assigning, actually weakens the person who claims it. We all have known patients who never move on from their beliefs that they are owed, that someone else has to fix them. Then, too, we may believe that claiming the role of victim and identifying a perpetrator is an attempt to seize power and attention from its rightful place. Sixty years ago, physical discipline of children was common in the home and in schools; now, a teacher can be fired for behavior that is a minor shadow of what used to happen. But what power remains to adults? And how are they to exercise it? These are questions that trouble all of us and on which there is little agreement. What is worse, our ideas are constantly changing, and evolving, so that today's standards are outmoded by tomorrow's.

A sociologist writing on the problem gives us an analogy from the psychotherapeutic process. Writing about post-traumatic stress disorder, and reflecting on the checkered history of social and professional understanding of child sexual abuse, starting with Freud, Bolen (4) states:

> The societal and professional response to child sexual abuse is . . . cyclical . . . with its phases of acceptance and suppression. Here, however, the more proper analogy may be one of posttraumatic stress disorder, with phases of intrusion and avoidance. The scope of the problem of child sexual abuse is, to a sophisticated society, an extreme threat to its self-perception. As such, the knowledge of the scope of child sexual abuse is proving exceptionally difficult to integrate. Just as the process of working through requires an acceptance of the shadow side of oneself, so does the societal process of accepting such an horrific shadow side. To expect and wish for an easy acceptance of this shadow side is idealistic. Those who watch their clients struggle to accept what they do not want to know about themselves, whether it is their victimization or their victimizing, know this truth. Being with clients who process knowledge about themselves, and sometimes about those

they love, requires the proper respect for their defenses, allowing them to avoid the truth until they build the internal fortitude to return to it. Ultimately, as clients cycle between intrusive and avoidant stages they also slowly integrate the knowledge into their being.

How can we expect anything less of a society that does not want to wear the label of a sexually violent society? (5)

I believe in this formulation. Our society both sensationalizes and ignores the questions of childhood trauma. We set up agencies to deal with it, underfund them, then publicly berate them when their inevitable imperfections surface. Articles on the front page fade quickly. We need a better understanding that this is everyone's problem. Further, we need an admission by everyone of the extent to which violence as a "solution" to all sorts of problems has permeated all our lives. We cannot just fault the professional schools. As medical professionals, however, I believe we have a special privilege and obligation to witness, to question, to synthesize and speak the truth, as best we understand it.

Childhood Sexual Abuse as One Example

The definition of childhood sexual abuse and, as referenced above, all abuse, is contextual, evolving, and subjective. In order to practice medicine, we have to come up with a working hypothesis. We also must accept that such a construct will evolve. Just as our concepts of how to treat tuberculosis or how to screen for breast cancer are continuously changing, so too will our definitions and responses to childhood violence. Most of us would agree that a father raping his teenaged daughter and forcing her sister to watch constitutes sexual abuse. What about a father noticing, and commenting with pleasure, and feeling slightly aroused by his daughter's developing womanhood? What if he communicates his arousal to her, inadvertently or not so inadvertently?

In health care, we are asked to respond to the human needs that evolve from such instances of questionable judgment and behavior. We need a "working definition" of child sexual abuse in particular, that we acknowledge may change, may be challenged and challengeable, and will certainly be flawed. (For now I will ignore the definitions of physical abuse and neglect.) Here are a few:

Sexual abuse is any non-consensual activity of a sexual nature, contact or non-contact, between an adult and a person under 18, or between two children when there is a four-year or greater age difference (6).

[S]exual abuse (is) an act perpetrated upon a child by a significantly older person with the intent to stimulate the child sexually and to satisfy the aggressor's sexual impulses (7).

The involvement of dependent, developmentally immature children and adolescents in sexual activities that they do not fully understand, to which they are unable to give informed consent, or that violate the social taboos of family roles (8).

Weaving through the definitions are the elements which cause problems for our previously abused adult patients. Sexual abuse informs a child violently that s/he is helpless, ignorant, unimportant, a tool for someone else's gratification, alone, and often mistaken in placing trust in those entrusted with her/his care, or strangers, or persons of the opposite, or same sex. The experience is wrenching, stimulating, and confusing. It is impossible for the child to understand, and causes disconnection with the child's developing sense of bodily integrity, self-confidence, trust in self and others, self-worth, and safety. Anatomically, there is growing evidence that it permanently changes the developing brain (9).

As clinicians, we can notice how many of our abused patients have disruptions in elements we take for granted in the health care relationship. We have been taught that if we act in certain professional ways, we will "earn trust"; that people can and will yield their body integrity to us by understanding "informed consent," and so forth. But experiences of childhood abuse may truncate, or wither, a developing person's ability to enter a level playing field in this respect. Our traumatized patients may not experience themselves or have the capacity to behave as fully functioning adults in this way. Furthermore, some of what the medical encounter asks of them, routinely, may appear consciously or unconsciously to be an invitation to return to the experience of abuse. In their minds, the rules of our offer to help define another abusive situation, repetition of which is, of course, terrifying. They will respond accordingly.

Just how many people in our society have grown up with childhood sexual abuse? Research into this question has been going on for 20–30 years. Not surprisingly, results are plagued by methodological issues. How was sexual abuse defined? Who was asking? What about the people who did not/could not recall their abuse (a common problem)? We have to resign ourselves to rough estimates. Surprisingly, however, for many of us these rough estimates are good enough. The numbers are huge. They are big enough that anyone in health care with a reasonably busy practice will encounter a survivor of child sexual abuse from once to five or six times **per day**.

Let's look at a few of the surveys.

In 1983, Russell conducted a randomly sampled community survey of over 900 women. Twenty-eight percent had had an unwanted **sexual contact experience** by the time they were 14, and 38% by the time they were 18 (10).

In 1994, Finkelhor suggested that 20% of the female population and 5%–10% of the male population were abused by the age of 18 (11).

In 1999, Bolen and Scannapieco (12), using 1997 data and accepting only studies they judged of moderate or better rigor, provided a meta-analysis estimating the prevalence of prior abuse in the female population as between 30% and 40%, and in the male population, 3%–13%, stating that the male number for methodological reasons was likely to be falsely low.

Whereas earlier studies emphasized intrafamilial abuse—father-daughter incest, sibling incest, abuse by relatives—more recent studies have categorized extrafamilial abuse as being by far the more common. Strangers, acquaintances, "friends" of the family, dates, teachers, doctors, nurses, psychologists, camp counselors, ministers, priests, childcare workers—all have been implicated as perpetrators. All of these have been reported to use violence, threats, coercion, secrecy, grooming techniques, and double lives to get and maintain sexual access to their victims.

It is hard to look at this research and maintain a sense of "normalcy" about life in America, to maintain a belief in our way of life, not to pick an argument or explode with rage or disbelief. Imagine, then, how hard it is for an abuse survivor to remember, to expect to be believed, respected, or integrated into the fabric of our medical care, if we do not admit, and resonate with, what is going on in our nation. Dr. Gilligan, in writing his book about violent men, gave us an example of how we might listen and understand. We can use his experience to help us pursue professional lives that begin to correct the wrongs that have been done. We owe it to our patients to create an environment which respects and accommodates their truth, rather than continuing to nullify or objectify it. Our patients need a safe, knowledge-based haven in which to begin to heal.

References

1. Gilligan J, *Violence: Reflections on a National Epidemic*, GP Putnam's Sons, 1996.
2. Committee on Health Care for Underserved Women, American College of Obstetricians and Gynecologists, "Adult manifestations of childhood sexual abuse," *International Journal of Gynecology & Obstetrics* 74: 311–320, 2001.

3. Cohn F, Salmon ME, and Stobo JF, eds., *Confronting Chronic Neglect, The Education and Training of Health Professionals on Family Violence*, National Academy Press, Washington DC, 2002.
4. Bolen RM, *Child Sexual Abuse, Its Scope and Our Failure*, pp. 12–18, Kluwer Academic/Plenum Publishers, 2001.
5. Bolen RM, *Child Sexual Abuse*, citing Olafsen et al., p. 38, 2001.
6. How W, private communication, 2007.
7. National Center for Child Abuse and Neglect: "Child sexual abuse: incest, assault and sexual exploitation." Special Report. United States Department of Health, Education and Welfare publication no. OHDS) 79: 30166, 1978.
8. Kempe CH: "Sexual abuse, another hidden pediatric problem": the 1977 C. Anderson Aldrich Lecture. *Pediatrics* 62: 382, 1978.
9. Siegel DJ, "An Interpersonal Neurobiology of Psychotherapy: The Developing Mind and the Resolution of Trauma," in Solomon MF and Siegel DJ (eds.) *Healing Trauma: Attachment, Mind, Body and Brain*, pp. 1–56, WW Norton, 2003.
10. Russell DEH, "The incidence and prevalence of intrafamilial and extra familial sexual abuse," *Child Abuse and Neglect* 7: 133–146, 1983.
11. Finkelhor D, "Current information on the scope and nature of child sexual abuse," *The Future of Children* 4(2): 31–53, 1994.
12. Bolen RM and Scannapieco M, "Prevalence of child sexual abuse: A corrective meta-analysis," *Social Service Review* 73(3): 281–313, 1999.

2
Disclosure

Now

Only this moment holds
the power we crave
the tiny dynamo, the atom
waiting to be split. The past,
however miserable or
heavenly, is last night's dream,
the future a curtain of mist.
Now is the builder of cities,
The composer of symphonies.
Now is the lover, the suicide,
the newborn. Now is the pen
to the paper, the knife to
the throat, the kiss on the lips. (1)

Introduction

Why do people tell each other anything? Conversely, what is gained by not telling another person about something? What are the goals and effects of each communication?

Telling our stories brings us closer. Stories make things more real—for the listener, for the teller. The listener may hear it for the first or the twenty-first time, each time a little differently. But the teller also hears herself talking—sometimes with belief, sometimes with the feeling that she has made it up. The story contains the description but can never be the reality. And if the reality seems unreal—or is felt to be unbelievable—the listener's listening may help ground the teller.

Telling a story may also allow needed change to begin. A good story often highlights contradictions: between the now and the then, the wished for and the actual, between what is believed in and what happened. Contradictions bring discomfort—and awareness of unease, in the context of a trusted relationship, may initiate change in the teller. For many people, including victims of trauma, change initially seems unwelcome. The familiar strikes us as more trustworthy than the unknown. Here again, non-judgmental listening can lend credence to new possibilities.

Not-telling keeps things "safely" the same, encapsulated, preserved. It forestalls a new point of view.

In my experience, the subject of abuse or neglect occurring long ago is not near the top of a patient's manifest concerns. People may have "forgotten" about it, underrated its importance, or judged it irrelevant. Often, they will find the personal disruption and shame involved in telling so unpleasant that they avoid it. Past negative experiences with sharing can frequently play a role, as well.

We, as providers, can help or hinder. Our gestures and facial expressions may speak of receptivity and openness, or their opposite. Attuned listening, with its implied readiness and encouragement, helps. Gaining knowledge of the problem and of our own histories and past responses to trauma are important. It takes time to build one's capacity to hear and bear the truth. All of these qualities, however, are salient to would-be tellers.

A patient's moving from silence to speaking, particularly if invited by the very being of the provider, changes everything: the patient, the provider, and all of the work to be done, together—yes, even and especially, the "medical" work.

As this book unfolds, I hope it will become clearer why patients and health care providers need to know about patients' past trauma. In this chapter, I'd like to explore more about the act of telling, how it happens, and what it does for health and for caring.

What's So Special about Talking about Trauma and Abuse

We deal with disclosures all the time. We take "histories of the present illness." People come and tell us about their bodies, their families, their worries and hopes. With varying difficulty and skill, we learn how to take a sexual history. Often, our patients are more ready to tell us about some subjects than we are ready to ask.

Communication about childhood mistreatment is different. For one thing, it may never before have occurred. No matter how distressing or life-changing events were as a child, many adults carry them in a very inward place. When such communication does happen, it often takes years to come about. It may be disguised, wordless, behavioral, intra-psychic, or present only in the psyche of the doctor. It is attached to strong feeling. Most abuse-related emotions are unpleasant, confusing, or both. Finally, these feelings may attach both to the present moment and to past events about which knowledge may be incomplete, often forever.

Learning about and living with the knowledge of a patient's abusive or neglectful past, I find, creates a kind of "shadow presence" on the problem list. It isn't like "diabetes" or "caring for aging parent." We can learn about these latter problems, discuss them in the present, update mutual knowledge, and co-strategize. When patients communicate about prior trauma, their feelings and defenses may create a "this-is-different" sense about what they say. Being sensitive and respectful toward this patient requires that we return to this information only when we sense that the patient is willing, and when we can take in their narrative as it is told, on their terms. What knowledge or guesses are shared end up hovering in and around subsequent encounters, mostly not directly engaged with but never going away, either. It's like a fog off the coastline, sometimes advancing, often retreating. The inhabitants (us with our patients) just live with it.

In this book I'll be talking about childhood trauma and its adult manifestations, with an emphasis, often, on sexual abuse. Some effects of childhood abuse and neglect are general and are germane no matter what specifically happened. Sexual abuse has particular features which differentiate it further.

When such abuse takes place, a child becomes a means to someone else's end. Regardless of the needs, age, readiness, or consent of the child, or the child's need for this person to function in other ways for his/her benefit, the child has been used to gratify the abuser's sexual—or other—desires. The abuse frequently takes place with coercion, or at least cajoling, and often ends with threats. Abusers threaten death, ostracism, ridicule, or removal of vital support. Sexual abuse is cloaked in secrecy, maintained with fear, and surrounded by confusion. Confusion also often ensues if the perpetrator is a beloved or needed individual. There is usually a grave power differential between perpetrator and victim. In addition, frequently a child's frightened, brave attempts to tell others about what has happened, despite these threats, are met with indifference, ridicule, blame, disbelief, and shunning. The truth is often perceived as dangerous to the integrity of the child's family system, or to our social system, and is treated accordingly.

Research on Disclosure

Social scientists have studied what happens when people talk about prior abuse, and the medical literature informs us.

In an interesting study of 41 adult Israeli survivors, Somer and Szwarcberg (2) looked at reasons all these people had waited years to disclose their abuse to anyone. They identified and later validated 10 personal psychological variables (e.g., "burden of the secret" or "mistrust of others"), five family-related variables (e.g., "loyalty," "concern for family integrity"), four social variables (e.g., "stigma," "media publicity"), and one trauma variable ("intensity"), which could either facilitate or delay disclosure by a victim. The researchers solicited for their research reasonably stable adults who were already in psychotherapy. A high percentage of those who were asked participated. Thirty-nine were women, two were men. Their ages ranged from 16 to 56. On average they had been abused for seven years in mid-to-late childhood. Although a substantial minority reported "always" knowing something was wrong, it took an average of six years, and in some cases decades, for each of these people to disclose to *anyone*. Furthermore,

> . . . in all cases but one, disclosure to the mother elicited a hostile/indifferent reaction; further, 95% of respondents chose to disclose to a nonfamily member. . . . [N]one of those who had disclosed during childhood perceived the disclosure as having had a positive impact on their lives (e.g., "The reaction I received silenced me until I was 46 years old."). The older the survivors were at the time of disclosure, the more likely they were to report an outcome positive for themselves. For example, 73% of those who first disclosed during adulthood felt the experience to be helpful to them (e.g., "I understood it wasn't my fault," or "It was only after the disclosure that I realized I deserved to heal.").

Personal variables which delayed disclosure included mistrust of others (including family), feelings of helplessness, and amnesia for the events. Social variables had an even stronger valence, the strongest being "fear of social rejection." Psychological abuse, (which had also occurred to over 90% of these clients), emotional neglect, and sexual abuse, in that order, were features of the abuse itself which delayed disclosure. Variables which tended to favor disclosure included media publicity, personal achievement, and altruistic concern for other victims.

Alaggia (3), again noting the 30%–80% of victims who delay disclosure until adulthood, argues for "expanded ways of defining and conceptualizing disclosure." She also suggests that disclosure may be a fluid process, rather than an event. Both of these have relevance to cases we will be discussing. She noted that "boys were less likely to disclose for varied reasons, including the increased risk of stigmatization attached to males' admitting to being victimized. The fact that boys are more often abused by males frequently raises associated fears of being labeled homosexual which, in a homophobic society, further prevents them from telling. . . . In addition, sexual exploitation of boys by older women is often mistakenly viewed as desirable and, therefore, their victimization is minimized or denied."

Using the Long Interview method, she studied 24 adult survivors—14 women, 10 men. All had suffered intra-familial abuse, and about one-third had endured extra-familial abuse, starting on average at age 6.5 years. Most abusers were men in a parent/grandparent role. Fifty-eight percent of these people had not disclosed until adulthood, and about half who did disclose before adulthood did so unintentionally. Some of them tried to disclose to the world as adolescents by acting out or expressing fears of family life—these acts were not understood or questioned, and therefore the communication failed in its intent. Half of those who waited did so because they had repressed memories, had forgotten what happened, or it happened so early in their life that they could not piece it together. Often, their memories were triggered by something: ". . . and it was like just like, one day, I had this huge flashback, and it was like (pause) at the end of one of the most severe incidents, and then I remember the last part when I was being cleaned up."

Alaggia concludes by noting that purposeful disclosure at any age is often met with skepticism ("Why didn't he tell sooner?" "How could she forget something so horrible?"). She argues for the need for trained professionals, alert to behavioral presentations, knowledgeable about fragmented stories and memories, and aware of the widespread existence and nature of child abuse.

None of the victims in either of these studies had first disclosed to a medical professional involved in the care of their lives and bodies, despite the potential intimacy and power of such an encounter.

Several studies discuss medical screening practices about child abuse. Generalists are reported to be relatively unlikely to ask (4,5,6). The majority felt they needed "more training" about asking and supporting survivors. On the other hand, a majority of women survivors in one study (7) were "relieved" or "hopeful" after disclosing, and "none reported feeling offended."

The American College of Obstetrics and Gynecology now recommends that its doctors screen every patient for a history of sexual abuse, and gives explicit guidelines about what to say (8). (By implication, practitioners are to use this knowledge in the care of patients.) In practice, perceived obstacles of limited time with patients, and a dearth of training, may limit many from opening this subject. White (9) details the positive effects of working with pregnant survivors to avoid traumatic stimuli during prenatal care and examinations, labor, delivery, and postpartum periods. She cites the positive effects of planning for the effects on survivors of being undressed, having the genital areas exposed, having invasive and at times painful examinations, and of labor and delivery itself.

A very interesting study by Seng et al. (10) qualitatively studied 15 women who had all had trauma histories and subsequently navigated a pregnancy. Pregnancy and delivery experiences were recollected. Through the interviews, women were divided into three groups: those who during pregnancy had been fairly far along in their recovery from abuse, those who were still at risk (experiencing trauma), and those who had been "not ready to know." For our purposes, we can contrast the first and third. Those who had already worked on recovery used the crisis of pregnancy as a vehicle for growth, seeking out knowledgeable providers and maintaining as much control over all facets of childbearing as they could. In contrast, those who had not yet achieved self-knowledge were still displaying their past trauma via symptoms, but they did not want open discussion of the trauma. They became passive, they dissociated, they compartmentalized. They were interested in having help with these issues but not with tracing them back to their cause. They described "knowing and not-knowing at the same time." "I kind of knew in some way it was affecting me, but I just couldn't connect the dots ever." It was best to have providers meet them at the level of their discomfort and symptoms. These women stressed that it was a process to move from coping by "not knowing" to being ready to name it, to acknowledge the long-term negative effects, and to take steps to improve their well-being. During their maternity care experience, they wanted their health care providers to name their evident distress, but not their abuse.

Friedman et al. (11) studied adult middle-class and working-class patients who both did and did not have abuse histories. The study took place in New England. Patients of both sexes and a variety of ages were recruited. Sixteen to seventeen percent at both sites had a history of physical and/or sexual abuse. Most had not been asked about it by their doctors, yet two-thirds to three-quarters of them felt they should be asked, and the vast majority felt their primary care doctors could help them if the response was positive. Of those who specifically did have a sexual trauma history, less than half said they would volunteer this history to their providers. Interestingly, those without a sexual trauma history were more likely to believe they would volunteer such information and were correspondingly less likely to favor a routine inquiry. A trauma history made people much more careful in their self-revelation.

Tener and Murphy (12) have reviewed over 30 years of literature on adult disclosure. They reiterated Alaggia's conceptualization of stages of revelation, testing the readiness and attitudes of the listener. Responses perceived as negative might shut the process down. They noted studies which described some survivors' emotional distance from their stories when first told (dissociation, see Chapter 4), or a boundary-less flooding of the listener—"vomiting" the story, in essence another way of distancing the teller from the story itself.

In their review, adult disclosers generally received more positive than negative responses, with a positive response described as "calm, supportive, and accepting, followed by encouragement to talk more about the abuse." Negative responses (which tellers do look for) included signs of discomfort, hostility, disbelief, dismissal, sexual arousal or interest in details by the listener, as well as giving in to the listener's emotions at the expense of the survivor's needs. Telling the story is a very difficult task.

A positive "being listened to" experience often resulted in emotional growth ("I was not to blame"), and a sense of healing. In contrast, not-telling, or delaying the telling, may result in negative symptoms and consequences of internalized stress, shame, and anger (12). Tener and Murphy concluded that "disclosure may serve to assist in the recovery process." They quote Baddeley and Singer (13): "The expression of a personal narrative to a listener is a powerful way in which we build our identities, forge interpersonal connections, and sustain a sense of purpose and meaning."

"If you are not part of the solution, you are part of the problem"

Certainly personal maturity, and the appearance of memories, are elements behind patients' disclosure over which we have little control. Nor do we have any control over the depth of trauma in a person's past, or what their family structure did or did not allow. However, from these studies we can infer how we might prepare ourselves to enable disclosure. Awareness of the steady drumbeat of violence in our society, and its effects, is certainly a prerequisite. We also need to work to be trustworthy and communicate pathways to personal power and strength. Most importantly, perhaps, we must remove stigma from the subject of violence and banish the fear of rejection which many survivors feel when they begin to remember and talk about what happened to them. The details of their experiences are abasing. Furthermore, perpetrators have often projected blame and guilt onto the child victims, and the adults they grow into live with an active sense of this guilt at many turns.

Shame, guilt, and fear may permeate a person's sense of self and invade their attempts to reveal themselves on any level—bodily, sexually, professionally, interpersonally—for decades, even a lifetime.

Skepticism about and ignorance of the effects of violence are often part of medical training. Only after shedding or accounting for these can a professional offer a survivor something more than a family member, or friend—that is, informed attitudes, and skills and resources which actually help rather than re-traumatizing patients, silencing them once again or causing them to lose faith in the profession.

Seng et al. (14) created a "Summary of participant messages to providers" after completing their small but deep qualitative study. These were framed in the context of obstetric practice but can be adapted to general practice, and to men and women both.

Desired Practices

In their summary, Seng and colleagues (14) suggest the following:

> ASK about abuse history, about how it is affecting her generally and in pregnancy, about what she needs from you, and, at each visit thereafter, ask truly open-ended questions and allow open time to discuss how she is doing with regard to post-traumatic stress concerns (e.g., "How are you?").
>
> ACKNOWLEDGE that trauma has long-term effects on some people, that she is not the only one, and that you are willing to work with her to address trauma-related needs or are able to refer her to a more appropriate provider.
>
> ASSESS repeatedly her risk for associated problems that are critical to perinatal outcomes: substance use, revictimization (current abuse), high-risk sexual practices, disordered eating, self-harm, postpartum mood and attachment disorders, and safety for her infant.
>
> ASSUME, in the absence of disclosure but in the presence of post-traumatic stress reactions, that the client could be a survivor and respond to her therapeutically but without forcing the issue.

AVOID triggering post-traumatic stress reactions by learning individual clients' triggers specifically and by increasing awareness of aspects of maternity care that are generally triggering (e.g., pelvic examinations, being touched without permission, feeling out of control).

ARRANGE more extensive contact that meets her needs via longer or more frequent visits with the main care provider or appointments with team members, and be ready to arrange connections to domestic violence programs, substance abuse treatment, or mental health services as appropriate.

ADVOCATE for appropriate program and financial resources to meet these clients' trauma-related needs, and consider using a secondary diagnosis of post-traumatic stress (or other appropriate related disorder) for clients who meet diagnostic criteria.

ASCERTAIN by follow-up of individuals and evaluation of practice over time whether trauma-related outcomes are being met in concert with perinatal goals.

Disclosure by a patient to a provider seems to require some safety within oneself and within a relationship. Once I own up to this, can I live with myself? Will others I love suffer harm? Once I speak it, can this person I am with bear to hear it without silencing, humiliating, or negating me? It takes some time to figure those things out. An abused child often becomes a wary, streetwise individual, and does not forget the lessons learned at the hands of his/her abuser(s).

As I hope is now obvious, it is really helpful if the provider, too, has done her homework. She needs to be alert, aware, to have personal, social, and professional resources about trauma, to be allowing without compelling, and understanding without overwhelming. Such readiness requires preparation.

There is another way of telling, to which we as physical health professionals have the "royal road," and that is the body and its maladies. The body is abused, the body feels, the body's nervous system encodes, the body remembers. With implicit memory (see Chapter 4), the meaning of an image or a feeling may not immediately be linked to an event, a psychic reality, or a piece of personal history. So, too, with "body memory." Connections may often be obscured, not obvious, confusing, disconnected. Over time, a symptom may develop a life and a voice of its own, speaking persistently but in code, so that neither we nor its sufferers, our patients, can understand what it is talking about. We both just know that it is commanding our attention.

I will speak more about the body and trauma in Chapter 7. For now, it is enough to realize that both straight-up conversation and physical symptoms can lead us into the memories of the past.

Nina

Nina first came to see me years ago in young middle age. Her primary care doctor was leaving the area and had in any case become inconvenient for her because of her own moves. She was concerned about being obese and about possibly being depressed, although she was not sure if her symptoms qualified. She had been overweight since her late teens and was engaged in an oft-repeated cycle of losing weight through a restricted calorie intake (unsupervised), only to regain it and more. She believed that any stress or change in her work/family life triggered her to eat compulsively. Most recently, she worked administering a community program and had begun to reflect on her own current symptoms of feeling "helpless, out of touch, and unable to utilize help of other people." In short, she was wondering about her own mental health.

In college, she alternated between dieting and compulsive overeating, which resulted in significant weight fluctuations. She had graduated from an excellent small school. Afterwards she entered and finished professional school and worked in business for a decade. Her cycle of weight loss/gain continued during her unhappy experience in graduate school, ultimately resulting in a weight gain of 40 pounds. A few years into her professional career she began to have panic attacks and, for the first time, she saw a therapist for a few sessions. Her weight at this point fluctuated up and down by 80 pounds. She disliked her profession and left it after 10 years. She had then begun working in community administration.

She was single, lived at times with various members of her family. She identified as lesbian but had no intimate relationship. She had been born and brought up in the United States, but in her latency years had moved with her family to another country, whose language she did not speak. Following their return, the family lived in several US cities, a fact she attributed to her father's "restlessness." Her parents eventually divorced.

History revealed one brief hospitalization for a sports-related injury during college. She was not a smoker, drinker, or user of drugs. When dieting, she exercised almost every day. During weight gain periods, she was relatively inactive. She had tended to have high cholesterol when her weight was up. There was a family history of high cholesterol.

She'd been sexually active with several women in the past. Now, she was in no relationship. "I am more interested in working on myself," she told me in that first meeting (twice). I wondered what work she sensed needed doing. Clearly, she was very overweight; she was also obviously highly intelligent but looked a little . . . what? Perplexed, clueless, ready, frightened? I was musing on her affect and my thoughts wandered. I don't know how Nina arrived at the subject of interpersonal violence, but that's when my attention snapped back to the present. I asked her if anything "like that" had ever happened to her. A look of amazed hopefulness came over her face, followed by a brief silence.

Nina told me that at the age of 11 or 12, while living abroad and walking home from a nearby swimming pool, she had been sexually assaulted by a neighborhood adolescent boy, who threatened to harm her if she told anyone. She remembered many of the details of the assault but nothing about what parts of her were penetrated. She did go home and tell her parents, the police were called, and she was seen by a doctor. But it was all done in a foreign language that she did not understand very well. She basically received only perfunctory care, and she and her family dealt with this by trying to forget about it and never discussing it. She had never had any effective therapy around it, and the one time she did see a therapist for the panic attacks, she never brought it up, nor did the therapist ask any relevant questions that might have prompted her to talk about it. She was put on Prozac quickly, had some trouble sleeping after two days, and stopped it.

Her physical exam was normal save for her weight and some mild exophthalmos.

A week or two later she returned and I administered the "Beck Depression Inventory," trying to get at the question of depression. Her mood, that day, was normal. "She is generally feeling more upbeat since our last conversation." She was interested in exploring herself further. I suggested she see a social worker with expertise in post- traumatic issues; that even though the rape occurred decades ago, its ramifications could be lingering. (Of course there would be other troubles as well.) She took the referral and sought treatment. She also decided to enroll in a medically supervised supplement-based weight management program at a nearby hospital, which other patients had attended with some success. Finally, she agreed to a colonoscopy and had this performed a few months later (normal).

After coming in for a cat bite, and a scalp neuritis, she was seen the next year for a general exam. She had done about six months of therapy with the social worker, who had suggested psychoanalysis. Nina declined; "I sense that (the therapist) was disappointed," she said. She was still thinking it over, however. (Was Nina disappointed?) She said she found the therapy helpful, without elaborating. She was "trying to get better" about her weight. After initial success in the hospital-based program, she had regained the weight over a period of time. Now, after rejoining the program, she had lost about eight pounds (she was again about 80 pounds overweight). Her home life and work life continued about the same. She was not in a partner relationship. Her exam was unchanged. I commented in my note (not to her) that she was "not interested in challenging the boundaries" at that moment.

Years passed. Struggles with weight continued. One year I wrote, her "family is irritable and angry": this contributed to her not eating a good breakfast. Often instead she would "treat herself" to a later, higher fat take-out breakfast, followed by deciding that the rest of the day was shot, food-wise, and that she should eat "whatever junk food she wants" . . . "try again tomorrow." She took on challenging jobs and worked long hours. She was in and out of the hospital-based, low calorie, supplement-based weight program at least three times, losing and then regaining 40–80 pounds. Her cholesterol was high when she was obese.

Further along, she had some counseling available to her through the weight loss program; she felt it was useless. Her mother had now developed breast cancer; there was a concern for genetic cancer syndrome in the family. Nina herself recently had had an abnormal mammogram, but a normal breast biopsy. She was awaiting BRCA testing on her mother and was sent to a genetic counselor to plan for her own screening.

At around the same time, she decided to "give up on weight programs." (She later returned.) She wanted and was given referrals to a new therapist. She did not wish to return to her old therapist. She saw the new therapist twice a month and, over time developed a romantic relationship with a woman with whom she moved away from the area for over a year. After the woman ended their sexual relationship and withdrew emotionally, Nina returned home, to our practice and to her old job. Now firmly in middle age, she began to think she might never be in a long-term relationship and had some equanimity with the thought. She had done some cognitive behavioral work (CBT) and came to firmly believe that "the rape was not my fault." She felt freed by this knowledge. She was back in weight management and was at her lowest weight in many years.

The Trajectory of Nina

Nina "spilled the beans" in our first encounter. Something about her appearance caused me to dissociate (Chapter 4)—her weight? her facial expression? I was brought back by her mentioning the word violence. With a direct question, she responded with her secret. Since then, she's been in and out of hiding. Perhaps her weight is her protection from vulnerability—gaining, losing in cycles. She has extraordinary discipline about losing it, and a helplessness or "fait accompli" about regaining. If I make even a small suggestion (about vulnerability, abuse, weight, whatever), she looks at me with amazed wonder.

I imagine her feelings: "This should have hurt but it didn't?" "How did you get in there?" I have always felt such potential lurking under her protective coat of fat.

More recently she took a major risk in trying life with a new partner, made some big life changes, found they did not work out, and came out of it not depressed or hopeless but instead with new insight and self-acceptance. She found the CBT program on her own and freed herself from a layer of blame she had not previously known was there.

Nina's strengths include curiosity about herself and bravery. She dared asking herself questions; she certainly took a leap in telling me what had happened. The power of her self-revealing, of the assault, and of her family's hiding from it (and her), was always sitting with us as we met. It permeated the interstices of her struggles with her weight. It undergirded her growth toward intimacy. It invited us to delve into it, or not, on each meeting. It required invitation (often secretively offered) from her, and intuition on my part, to go there. I hope that our interchanges gave her some strength and desire to proceed.

Gabe

Gabe's fuller story appears in the chapter on dissociation (Chapter 4). I'll present his journey to disclosure in brief here to see what we can learn.

Several decades ago, Gabe first came for general medical care. Fairly recently married, he was working while also in school at night. He complained of toenail fungus, of occasional episodes of proctalgia fugax, dating back 13 years, and of some innocent spots on his scrotum. When asked about exercise, told me he was a "pathetic lump." In fact, he was charming, earnest, and impishly humorous. He captivated me. Perhaps this is why I neglected to pay attention to his clues.

On reviewing family history, he told me that his parents had been divorced for over a decade. His father was currently having memories of child sexual abuse at the hands of his own father, Gabe's grandfather. I noted that this was painful for Gabe, who had, as a child, adored his grandfather.

I ask myself now what I might have done differently in this encounter. His symptoms center around his sexual organs. His self-concept (humorously and lightly expressed) was the opposite of the dominant culture's male ideal. And the current family drama—always intertwined and so useful as we explore the family history of disease—centered around the memories of sexual abuse. I could have taken note of this, as trauma can certainly be trans-generationally transmitted. It also has a way of being re-enacted through the generations, particularly when vigorous steps are not taken, and help given, before a person reaches his generative years.

I enjoyed this interesting story and even more Gabe's elegant, witty style, hinting at more to come. But—not revealing. That was for me to decide, and it never crossed my mind. If it had, I think now that I might not have tried to probe any of his physical presentation, but I might have tried to get him to talk more about what happened to his father and his grandfather, as they are in the "someone else" category, less threatening to Gabe's sense of who he himself is. Somewhere in the charting, I would have stowed a note about "genital concerns" and just waited.

More genital concerns, and more stories came over the years, without enlightenment. Perhaps you, like me, sometimes get a creepy sense when a client repeatedly focuses on sexuality or sex organs. This did not happen with Gabe and me, because of his earnestness and his ability to tell a great story. But the creepy sense is a clue; and it must be handled with great respect—for the clue, and even more for your patient. Perhaps your patient is compelled by forces within to focus "too much attention" on sexuality. Sitting right next to this compulsion are our familiar companions—guilt and shame.

Example: a not so recent newspaper article (15) detailed the possible solving of a case of repeated rapes over a number of years in a nearby community. Evidence had finally pointed to a local construction worker, a somewhat isolated man who was nevertheless respected by his co-workers as skilled and reliable, always in a good mood. When police arrived in daylight on the building scene to confront and arrest him, he began openly weeping before they even got out of their cars. That was what struck his shocked colleagues—his breakdown into uncontrolled tears.

Here's the event that broke things open for me and Gabe, years into our relationship. He presented to me one week after a urethral hemorrhage which occurred during lovemaking. He had bled copiously; his wife called 911, and he'd gone to the ER, where bleeding slowed and stopped on its own, and he was sent home. He did not require transfusion.

In discussing the event and trying to decide what to do, further history emerged. Gabe was and had been for years quite sexually active, stimulating himself to orgasm often several times daily. He had been abstinent, out of fear, for the week since the hemorrhage, and told me "I am going a little crazy"—which, delivered in his well-brought up way, I took as an understatement of his condition.

It took more time to understand the context for his strong sexual drive. It involved an entire rearrangement of his understanding of his family of origin, and ways in which he had been used to shore up his parents' needs, thwarted desires, and coping mechanisms. (For more on this and what we can learn, please see Chapter 4.) For now, we can understand that it was Gabe's body, like Nina's, that "spoke" about his trauma to me, as his physician. In both cases, too, there were prior verbal and behavioral clues that sometimes I caught, and many times did not. I present these cases as examples to help fellow clinicians to hear what is and is not being said, beneath the words that our patients speak.

The Importance of Disclosure

Disclosure about prior, or ongoing, trauma brings about fear and shame, anxiety and dismay. It may also, if properly understood and handled, widen, deepen, and change both the doctor–patient relationship and the work that is to be done within, and outside of, that relationship.

As I've already mentioned in Chapter 1, and will elaborate on in chapters to come, abuse and neglect alter the whole being of its victims. Clients with trauma histories are more prone to a wide variety of health problems broadly understood as "diseases of stress." These diseases exist in body and mind together. Part of their treatment is the amelioration, to the extent possible, of the burdens currently placed on patients by their traumatic past.

A disclosure about abuse may signal a level of trust achieved, a powerful readiness to grow on the part of the client, a problem with boundaries, an unconscious "blurt," or even a mistake. A careful evaluation of the state of the client after such an event is in order. You have been entrusted with a secret, the telling of which is often very difficult and whose ramifications are complex. Care and respect for the patient and the problem are in order. Integration of this knowledge by you may take time.

Since there is such stigma in our society about childhood abuse, I recommend putting the information obtained into the chart, and identifying the past abuse as a separate but vitally related health problem, to be returned to, or not, in a variety of ways in the future. Otherwise, we, like our patients, can forget about the trauma or minimize it. This is precious information, hard-won by both doctor and patient, and it must not be wasted. In addition, your patient may need repeated affirmation, or other signals of "positive regard" whenever the subject comes up.

How you and your patient will use this information will vary with the individuals involved. It can be as simple or complex as needed, as deep as you and your client want to go, and as divergent and inflected as both of you yourselves are. This is part of the inherent richness of general medicine.

References

1. Kessenich L, *Age of Wonders*, Big Table Publishing, 2016.
2. Somer E and Szwarcberg S, "Variables in delayed disclosure of childhood sexual abuse," *American Journal of Orthopsychiatry* 71(3): 332–334, 2001.
3. Alaggia R, "Many ways of telling: expanding conceptualizations of child sexual abuse disclosure," *Child Abuse and Neglect* 28(11): 1213–1227, 2004.
4. Lee A, Coles J, Lee S, and Kulkarni J, "Primary healthcare practitioners' screening practices and attitudes towards women survivors of child abuse," *Mental Health and Family Medicine* 9(3): 181–189, 2012.
5. Friedman LS, Samet JH, Roberts MS, Hudlin M, and Hans P, "Inquiry about victimization experiences, a survey of patient preferences and physician practices," *Archives of Internal Medicine* 152: 1186–1190, 1992.
6. Neher JO, "The decade dance," *Annals of Family Medicine* 3(5): 462–463, 2005.
7. Lee A, Coles J, and Kulkarni J, "Women survivors of child abuse—don't ask, don't tell," *Australian Family Physician* 41(11): 903–906, 2012.
8. Committee on Health Care for Underserved Women, "Adult manifestations of childhood sexual abuse," *Obstetrics and Gynecology* 118: 392—395, 2011.
9. White A, "Responding to prenatal disclosure of past sexual abuse," *Obstetrics and Gynecology* 123(6): 1344–1347, 2014.
10. Seng JS, Sparbel KJH, Low LK, and Killion C, "Abuse-related posttraumatic stress and desired maternity care practices: women's perspectives," *Journal of Midwifery and Women's Health* 47(5): 360–370, 2002.
11. Friedman LS et al., "Inquiry about victimization experiences," 1992.
12. Tener D and Murphy SB, "Adult disclosure of child sexual abuse: a literature review," *Trauma, Violence, and Abuse* 16(4): 391–400, 2015.
13. Baddeley JL and Singer JA, "A social interactional model of bereavement narrative exposure," *Review of General Psychology* 13, 202–218, 2009.
14. Seng JS, et al., "Abuse-related posttraumatic stress," 2002.
15. Allen E, Schworm P, and Ellement JR, "Suspect arrested in rapes," *The Boston Globe*, October 22, 2015.

3

Post-Traumatic Stress Disorder

Not in shyness but in disgust
the owl
turns its face from me and pours itself
into the air, hurrying

until it is out of sight—
and, after all,
even if we came by some miracle
upon a language which we both knew,

what is it I might say
there in the orange light of early morning,
in the owl's resting time
that would have any pluck and worth in it?—

not admonition, or blame,
and not recrimination,
and not, I say, unholy weeping,
and not, for god's sake, any bending of the knees

in the cold and rough grass
under its gold and glassy eyes
which, in such a conversation, you must imagine
turned upon you . . . (1)

Introduction

In many areas of life, trauma survivors inhabit a different world than other people. They have been a witness to and/or recipient of cruel and senseless behavior at the hands of seen and unseen others. They have experienced powerlessness, weakness, their ability to be used for others' benefit. Such life events evoke feelings of terror, rage, shame, and hopelessness. Such events are also felt to be "unspeakable" in ordinary civil discourse, and often they are not spoken of.

If people survive their encounter or encounters with "the worst," some emerge changed and unable to recover. Their thoughts, sensations, behavior, and emotions become more negative, constricted, fearful. They begin to behave in ways that neither they nor others understand. Ultimately, both the nature of the trauma and its effects on people isolate those that are changed in this way.

In this chapter, we will examine post-traumatic stress disorder, its history, definitions, and manifestations. We will review some of what is known about the brain and PTSD. We will discuss why some get it, and some do not. We will review how it may manifest in the course of clinical care, and how we might best respond.

PTSD Defined

Ten to thirty percent of people develop PTSD after a shock or injury. Most people who live through a trauma will have an *acute* trauma reaction consisting of (a) unwanted reliving of memories of the trauma, (b) acting out of the trauma in dream life, and (c) sudden feelings of dread and horror. If, after one month, these and other symptoms have not cleared, one is considered to have developed a more chronic derangement known as post-traumatic stress disorder (PTSD) (2).

According to *DSM V* (2013), a diagnosis of PTSD involves five criteria and two qualifiers.

A. Exposure to actual or threatened death, serious injury, or sexual violence in one (or more) of the following ways:
    1. Directly experiencing the traumatic event(s).
    2. Witnessing in person, the event(s) as it occurred to others.
    3. Learning that the traumatic events(s) occurred to a close family member or close friend. In cases of actual or threatened death of a family member or friend, the event(s) must have been violent or accidental.
    4. Experiencing repeated or extreme exposure to aversive details of the traumatic event(s) (e.g., first responders collecting human remains; police officers' repeated exposure to details of child abuse).

In this volume, we are talking about childhood abuse and neglect. However, PTSD is a generic syndrome which occurs equally to rape victims and war veterans, to survivors of motor vehicle accidents, and to children molested by neighbors.

B. Presence of one (or more) of the following intrusion symptoms associated with the traumatic event(s), beginning after the traumatic event(s) occurred:
   1. Recurrent, involuntary, and intrusive distressing memories of the traumatic event(s).
   2. Recurrent distressing dreams in which the content and/or affect of the dream are related to the traumatic event(s).
   3. Dissociative reactions (e.g., flashbacks) in which the individual feels or acts as if the traumatic event(s) were recurring. (Such reactions may occur on a continuum, with the most extreme expression being a complete loss of awareness of present surroundings.)
   4. Intense or prolonged psychological distress at exposure to internal or external cues that symbolize or resemble an aspect of the traumatic event(s).
   5. Marked physiological reactions to internal or external cues that symbolize or resemble an aspect of the traumatic event(s).

In this latter category would be included such things as tachycardia, piloerection, sweating, and perhaps vasodepressor reactions.

C. Persistent avoidance of stimuli associated with the traumatic event(s), beginning after the traumatic event(s) occurred, as evidenced by one or both of the following:
   1. Avoidance of or efforts to avoid distressing memories, thoughts, or feelings about or closely associated with the traumatic event(s).
   2. Avoidance of or efforts to avoid external reminders (people, places, conversations, activities, objects, situations that arouse distressing memories, thoughts or feelings about or closely associated with the traumatic event[s]).

D. Negative alterations in cognitions and mood associated with the traumatic event(s), beginning or worsening after the traumatic event(s) occurred, as evidenced by two (or more) of the following
   1. Inability to remember an important aspect of the traumatic event(s) (typically due to dissociative amnesia and not to other factors such as head injury, alcohol, or drugs).

2. Persistent and exaggerated negative beliefs or expectations about oneself, others, or the world.
3. Persistent, distorted cognitions about the cause or consequences of the traumatic event(s) that lead the individual to blame himself/herself or others.
4. Persistent negative emotional state (e.g., fear, horror, anger, guilt, or shame).
5. Markedly diminished interest or participation in significant activities.
6. Feelings of detachment or estrangement from others.
7. Persistent inability to experience positive emotions (e.g., inability to experience happiness, satisfaction, or loving feelings).

E. Marked alterations in arousal and reactivity associated with the traumatic event(s), beginning or worsening after the traumatic event(s) occurred, as evidenced by two (or more) of the following:
1. Irritable behavior and angry outbursts (with little or no provocation), typically expressed as verbal or physical aggression toward people or objects.
2. Reckless or self-destructive behavior.
3. Hypervigilance.
4. Exaggerated startle response.
5. Problems with concentration.
6. Sleep disturbance (e.g., difficulty falling or staying asleep, or restless sleep).

F. Duration of the disturbance . . . is more than one month.

G. The disturbance causes clinically significant distress or impairment in social, occupational, or other important areas of functioning.

H. The disturbance is not attributable to the physiological effects of a substance (e.g., medication, alcohol) or another medical condition (3).

Susan

Susan came to the clinic with feelings of depression, and less interest than usual in her daily activities. In addition to worrying about her daughter's upcoming divorce and well-being, she and her family had just lived through a terrifying event six weeks prior. She, her daughter, and two grandchildren had been vacationing on a remote island where the family had a primitive cabin. A forest fire began in a patch of forest close to the cabin. They were alone on the island. The fire eventually grew into an area "the size of a room in a house."

Susan called a number, hanging by the phone, for forest fires. The number was out of date. She then called 911 and called some other locals on the nearby mainland. Her daughter tried to put out the fire with buckets of water from the lake. Doing so, she sprained her ankle, panicked and told the children to start packing. One of the children tried to get the outdoor pump working, but it was broken. The other child started packing. Susan, feeling responsible for everyone, did not think the hose would reach the fire, but used a rug to keep the fire from spreading. Finally, she remembered that there were local volunteer firemen to call. They came, extinguished the fire, and saved the house.

Susan now reported feeling listless, depressed, and pessimistic. She blamed herself for not organizing everyone's response better. She worried one grandchild was permanently traumatized. She couldn't figure out why she hadn't called the firefighters earlier. She felt guilty that the household had not been prepared for a fire. She kept going over her thoughts and decisions at the time. She was having terrible troubles getting to sleep and staying asleep. Images of the fire, the house, and her daughter's state crowded her mind.

Susan was having an acute stress reaction and early PTSD. Her doctor listened to the whole story, feeling some of everyone's fear. She, a fellow first-born, imagined Susan's sense of responsibility and failure both. The two parsed through the intensity and difficulty of the decisions and reactions the patient had had, and the doctor tried to lessen some of her self-blame. Susan was encouraged to discuss this event with others not in her family, picking wisely and widely, letting people know, particularly, how she had felt. Susan's doctor gave her a small amount of zolpidem for the short term, to improve sleep onset.

Six weeks later, Susan reported that her depression and self-blame had lifted, she was sleeping normally off medication, and she was no longer preoccupied by memories of the event and her reactions.

Susan had short-term, time-limited PTSD which responded to attuned listening, to sharing (repeatedly) her emotions at the time of the event, and to reframing some of her thoughts, as well as specific symptom management.

Complex PTSD

It is important to know how to handle people's acute trauma reactions. The patients that concern us in this book are likely to have much more resistant and persistent symptoms—ones laid out in the *DSM 5* explication above, and ones that are long-lasting. These symptoms have woven themselves into a person's way of being. In addition, some in the mental health field are working with an as-yet-unsanctioned (by DSM) diagnostic category known as "complex PTSD" or "Disorders of Extreme Stress, not otherwise specified" (DESNOS). This category refers to clients who have lived through *inescapable,* repetitive episodes of trauma, often lasting years, often at a young or not fully mature age. Seven criteria have been proposed (4) for this category, with the prior trauma understood as a requirement for the diagnosis, as in the American Psychological Association's definition:

1. *Alterations in regulation of affective impulses,* including difficulty with modulation of anger and self-destructiveness. (This requirement refers to the overwhelming nature of negative affect and consequent behaviors we see in this group of clients).
2. *Alterations in attention and consciousness,* leading to amnesias and dissociative episodes and depersonalization. (This criterion emphasizes more severe dissociative responses and diagnoses than does the 2013 category B, above).
3. *Alterations in self-perception,* such as a chronic sense of guilt and responsibility, and ongoing feelings of intense shame. (Often this group of clients feels damaged, different at their core, defective, taking on *as identity* some of what their perpetrators have said about them or to them, for instance).
4. *Alterations in perception of the perpetrator,* including taking on the perpetrator's views, or feeling a sympathetic bond with the perpetrator . . . .(Some clients will rationalize their perpetrator's behavior, or identify with him/her—carrying impulses to behave in a similar fashion, for instance).
5. *Alterations in relationship to others* (e.g., pervasive distrust, or not being able to feel intimate with others). These problems will extend to the doctor–patient relationship, as well as relationships with the health care system in general.
6. *Somatization and/or medical problems* that relate directly to the type of abuse suffered and resultant physical damage, or that diffusely involve all body symptoms. (This is a category very important to us as physical medicine providers).
7. *Alterations in systems of meaning,* including hopelessness about finding anyone who can help or understand one's suffering, and despair of being able to recover. (Often people's spiritual lives are deeply damaged in complex PTSD. People lose their belief in God, in the goodness of others, in the idea of a society organized for the safety of its citizens.)

Briere, Scott, and Jones (5) note the paradoxical lack of some of the symptoms of PTSD in this delineation of complex PTSD. In particular, they comment on the absence of some symptoms in categories B, C, or E in the 2013 definition (intrusive, avoidant, arousing). I understand some of this to reflect the fact that by definition, those who have what Herman and others are describing have had *repetitive* episodes of trauma during times of *developmental immaturity and vulnerability*. Avoidant behavior over time may lead to "alterations in relationship to others." Arousal phenomena awaken the hypothalamic-pituitary axis and involve the autonomic nervous system, which may be precursors for persistent somatic symptoms and disease.

Familiarity with both definitions is needed to comprehend both what we see our trauma patients experiencing and how they behave. People may present to us with self-destructive addictions, with chronic illnesses toward which they have developed attitudes of "learned helplessness," with resistant pain or weakness without obvious cause, or with social isolation and loneliness. Any of these may reflect the existence of PTSD, complex or not, and its antecedent in trauma, neglect, dependency, and inescapability. In this chapter we will work within the frameworks of both definitions.

Clyde

While attending on the general medical wards some years ago, after a week of work together the resident suggested at the end of rounds that one intern present a patient to me with whom he was struggling. "See what she says about *him*," he said. Clyde was a man in his 60s with a serious infection; he had recently left a neighboring institution (where care for the same problem was underway) against medical advice. "He always ends up coming here," noted the intern with an attitude of despair. Clyde was diabetic, could no longer see well, and had had an above-the-knee amputation on one leg. He was a registered sex offender. He frequently disrupted his own care, pulling out IVs and refusing treatments. He was going to require long-term intravenous medications but did not have a home setting where he could receive these. He had no family or friends who were suitable caregivers, as all had social and behavioral issues of their own. He needed to go to a skilled nursing facility, but he only wanted one in particular, as he felt the others treated him poorly. (He had been to many of them already in his life.) The dilemma, as perceived by the intern, was how to care for him in the face of his self-defeating, uncooperative actions and his resource-limiting behaviors.

I suggested this new doctor start by admitting Clyde's loathsome status as a violator of the social compact. In so doing I tried to help him admit and get comfortable with his own disgust with his patient's conduct, and dismay at his "bad luck" at becoming his primary caregiver for a period of time that seemed to be extending indefinitely. In addition, I suspected the intern was beginning to realize that this would not be the last time he had to care for someone for whom he had negative feelings. I wonder if he had anticipated this, in choosing medicine as a career. I certainly had not, at his age. I suggested that he commend himself, daily, just for going into the patient's room. He could also work on finding some basis for liking his patient, some neutral but mutually enjoyable ground, such as humor, sports, or a shared interest (the intern had already done this on his own). I suggested that he was in a position to find out what the patient's goals were and work from there, as opposed to trying to impose the medical system's goals upon the patient. I encouraged him to remember that Clyde was not born a sex offender, but had had experiences, likely very traumatic ones, that "taught" him in ways he had not yet shared with his young doctor, nor even yet, perhaps, with himself.

The patient went on to be rejected by all skilled nursing facilities. One day, the intern reported, the patient cried, sharing his despair at being unwanted by anyone. I asked this young doctor if the patient's tears felt to him like genuine grief. The intern noted that they had. Furthermore, this young doctor was able to sit with him while Clyde grieved.

As the weeks went by, the intern developed a kind of tending, if not tender, protective relationship with Clyde, worrying that some specialist's treatment recommendations might be dangerous for him given his lifestyle after discharge, and wondering how to disagree with his superiors to advocate for a safer program. At the same time, he was intermittently wary about possible negative side effects of his being Clyde's primary provider, worrying about the patient's potential for blaming his misfortunes, past and likely forthcoming, on the medical system, including this intern. We discussed, repeatedly, the power of the informed consent process and of concise but complete documentation as a protection against the vagaries of patient complaints. Ultimately the patient was discharged home, this particular disease eradicated.

This patient, losing parts and functions to various illnesses while still in middle age, did not "carry" the diagnosis of complex PTSD, but the intern was living its effects with him. No one in the hospital knew anything of the patient's early life history. But Clyde had problems with affect regulation, self-destruction, trust, progressive physical deterioration, and, at his core, hopelessness about his state. His hopelessness and associated cynicism, his fear and shame, carried over to his treatment team. My challenge, as the team's guide for the month, was to sort out what was happening for the young treating physicians, work with them on relationship formation and on how to proceed with a viable plan, and help them understand how to take care of themselves while caring for the patient. We shall return to these tasks later in this chapter.

Biological Substrates of PTSD

Post-traumatic stress disorder has been characterized variably as a disorder of anxiety, of dissociation, of somatization, and of personality, though it does not fit neatly into any of these categories and encompasses some of all. Thinking biologically, we could also define it as a disorder of altered neuroendocrine function, or even a disorder of memory. The past several decades have brought much research on brain structure and function in many mammalian species, including humans. We can study humans in various states due to the advent of volumetric MRI studies and functional MRI resonance scanning. There is an enormous literature in this area, and I refer interested readers to excellent summaries written elsewhere (6). My goal in this section is simply to impart the idea that trauma in early life changes brain structure and function going forward. Our patients with PTSD (as well as depression, dissociation, anxiety, etc.) because of childhood abuse and neglect function with nervous systems that have diminished capabilities, and unsettled regulatory systems.

The stress response, which involves the hypothalamic-pituitary axis, is among the most studied of these subjects. It can be studied in a wide variety of mammals whose physiology in this regard is close enough to humans that we can postulate some basic theories about how we humans work. Mammals have been studied in various stages of development, creating the basis for understanding age-related vulnerabilities of the central nervous system (CNS). Humans, for ethical reasons, have been studied as adults, when they can consent.

A stressful event may be perceived by any of a number of sensory systems in the brain. They in turn route information via the thalamus and amygdala to the hypothalamus and the locus ceruleus, among others. The medial paraventricular nucleus of the hypothalamus contains high concentrations of corticotropin release factor (CRF), which when released stimulates the anterior pituitary to release adrenocorticotropic hormone (ACTH), which stimulates the human adrenal to release cortisol. Interestingly, CRF also seems to be a neurotransmitter in the amygdala, a part of the temporal lobe involved in emotional processing (especially fear), and in areas of the brainstem which regulate the locus ceruleus and the median raphe nuclei, which contain dense amounts of norepinephrine and serotonin, respectively. Thus CRF release can, via the brainstem activity, stimulate the adrenergic portions of the adrenal as well as directly releasing norepinephrine into the system, causing adrenergic autonomic arousal. In addition, there is evidence that CRF release impacts behavioral control and immune function in the whole organism.

Studies in various mammals using models of developmental stress, such as periods of maternal deprivation, have shown that after these animals mature, their stress responses have changed compared to controls. For instance, rats with periods of early life maternal deprivation have enhanced ACTH and cortisol-like responses to various stressors. In addition, their subsequent behavior is affected: they seemed to enjoy less, explore less, and startle more, at the same time having evidence of increased CRF transmission. Nemeroff states:

> Taken as a whole, longer periods of maternal separation induce the development of symptoms that resemble mood and anxiety disorders. . . . Although the data extrapolated from animal studies to patients with psychiatric disorders must be interpreted with some caution, preclinical findings suggest that there is a critical period during development when the consequences of stress lead to long-term neurobiological changes, most prominently alterations of the CRF neural circuits, that increase vulnerability for development of mood and anxiety disorders in response to subsequent stressor exposure in later life.
>
> Studies in adult humans with histories of trauma have noted similar changes in the setpoint of stress response. For instance, studies in abused women have shown increased daily cortisol excretion, and elevated ACTH and cortisol responses to stressful (laboratory) situations, over that of controls without childhood stress (7).

Lanius et al. (8) have reviewed some of what has been conceptualized and observed in brain research recently in people both with and without PTSD.

They begin with the concept of different "layers" of brain: reptilian, limbic, and neocortical. The first concerns itself with arousal, autonomic function, and reproduction—basic species survival. The limbic system, or the emotional brain, concerns itself with emotion, memory, learning. The neocortex enables speech, thought, self-awareness, and allows, via the corpus callosum, communication between the two hemispheres, which have very different functions. The neocortex is the part of the brain which distinguishes human beings from the rest of the animal kingdom.

Each of these parts can perceive, and interact with, the outside environment. They also interact with each other, with a human response to anything comprised of a mixture of activities of these layers of the brain. The thalamus, which is positioned between the first two levels of brain, is hypothesized to be the receiving center for almost all sensory information (except smell!), and the relay center for such information to all parts of the brain. Thalamic dysfunction, which has been observed in subjects with PTSD (9,10) may account for the existence of "sensory fragments" in that disorder—sensory experiences and memories unattached to a cohesive story about what happened.

In subjects with PTSD, there is also evidence for a disturbance in lateralization of brain function. During recall of traumatic memories, subjects without PTSD have more brain activity in their left hemispheres, while those with PTSD have more in their right. It is speculated that this is because traumatic memories in those who develop PTSD actually involve different neural networks. Experimentally, the brains of those without PTSD "showed brain activation patterns consistent with verbal episodic memory retrieval" with "greater levels of brain activation in the left prefrontal areas." Compare this with the PTSD patients who "showed more activation in the right posterior areas" . . . showing "patterns of neural activation associated with much more non-verbal patterns of memory retrieval." It is speculated that this right brain, non-verbal memory storage may be the neural basis for sensory-based flashbacks often experienced by those with PTSD. These flashbacks, along with other phenomena, in turn govern behavior, response to the environment, perception of others, thoughts, and worldview.

Parenthetically, Schore (11) and others have advocated interpersonal treatment of patients with PTSD based in part on this right brain dominance. Specifically, he describes treatment involving right brain to right brain communication between sufferer and treater, perhaps another way of understanding transference and countertransference.

Lanius et al. go on to delineate brain areas thought to be involved in the neural mechanisms underlying traumatic experience. These include:

the *amygdalae* (right and left), involved in "fear conditioning" and perhaps in freezing

the *medial prefrontal cortex*, which inhibits the limbic system, including the amygdalae, and is part of cognitive processing and memory retrieval, and perhaps, stress modulation

the *anterior cingulate gyrus*, which is extensively connected with cortical and subcortical structures, and plays some role in awareness of emotions and in linking body and behavior

the *hippocampus*, like the amygdalae, is part of the temporal lobe connecting amygdalae and cortex, involved in memory and vulnerable to chronic stress, with shrinkage and death observed in combat veterans and adult women survivors of childhood sexual abuse. Notably (and see below), some feel this anatomic abnormality might pre-exist and predispose people to the development of PTSD—not be the result of it. Either way—there are suggestions that this may be partially reversible with treatment.

the *insula*, located in the medial frontal and parietal lobes, under the temporal wings, "preferentially involved in the emotional response to potentially distressing cognitive stimuli, interceptive sensory stimuli, and body sensations." Notice how it may potentially receive input from all three levels of brain. Some have hypothesized that the right insula in particular is the anatomic basis for "knowing how one feels." Researchers have noted differences in pathways of insular activation between subjects with PTSD and dissociation, and those without it. Those with the former "reported feeling removed from their own bodies as well as from the emotional content of the traumatic memory." Again, this is evidence that the brain functions differently in these subjects. Finally,

the *orbitofrontal cortex*, tucked under the frontal lobes just over the eyes, is another area highly connected to other cortical and subcortical parts of the brain, and positioned to receive "a wealth of information about what is happening in the environment and what plans are being organized by other cortical areas." It is connected to systems of autonomic arousal and control. It is an area highly sensitive to the quality of the caregiver/infant relationship, and vulnerable to faulty maturation in infancy and toddlerhood due to abuse/neglect in that relationship, leading to strength or weakness in the processing of emotional information, body regulation, and coping with stress. This area may be where the "attachment system" sits.

Lanius et al. point out the different nature of subjectively experienced traumatic memories in those with PTSD and those without. Whereas people without PTSD "recall their traumatic memory as a memory of the past, a normal autobiographical memory," those with it have instead a "nonverbal pattern." This pattern consists of "activation of the occipital lobes, right parietal lobe, and posterior cingulate gyrus" and result in "timeless, intrusive sensory fragments that often cannot be expressed as a narrative." Subjects without PTSD "activate neural networks more consistent with verbal patterns of memory retrieval . . . left prefrontal cortex and anterior cingulate."

Finally, as noted in our first definition, the same traumatic event may produce a syndrome of PTSD with hypo-arousal (numbing, distancing), or one with intrusive thoughts and dreams, or both –or no PTSD at all, depending on many factors. Why this might be so will be the subject of our next inquiry.

Risk Factors for PTSD

Not everyone gets PTSD after a traumatic event. In fact, the majority of humans are sturdy or resilient enough that they "get on with it" after processing such a major event in their own way. Efforts have been made to understand what characterizes those who don't or can't "get over it," and we know something more about this than we did 10 or 20 years ago. Correlates within the development of PTSD can help us understand how we are to care for those who have it. We must note that all this research is fraught with methodologic problems of many types. We don't even know yet what we don't know.

Elements of the abuse itself are linked to PTSD likelihood and severity. Sexual abuse—both childhood and that experienced in adulthood—is the human trauma most likely to induce PTSD. Childhood survivors of prolonged abuse—for instance, those raised in Satanic cults—may be worse off than those who have experienced one or two events, such as harassment or indecent exposure. Similarly, both the duration and severity of abuse—the amount of distortion in reality, the apparent threat to life/safety, the cruelty involved, the amount of physical harm done—are linked to the more likely formation of a complex post-traumatic stress disorder (12).

The nature of the victim's family and social relationships at the time of the abuse may predict the development of PTSD. Whether or not the perpetrator was a family member, family instability, or a family history of mental symptoms, including anxiety or disordered mood, are in some studies positively linked its development after trauma (13).

Since Bowlby's first studies on the nature of human attachment (14) were published, an enormous amount of work has gone into defining and studying the nature and effects of different types of attachment relationships occurring between primary caregivers (often, but not always, mothers) and their infants. We will discuss attachment and its ramifications further in Chapter 8. It is clear, however, that a "secure" attachment in early life provides a buffer against trauma; such relationships are marked by emotional mutuality, both stimulation and calming at appropriate times, repair by the caregiver when misattunement occurs, and growth and maturation, particularly of right brain functions, in the infant. Such a relationship provides the basis for appropriate trust, emotional intelligence, and self-regulation and soothing later in life. It also provides a defense against the development of PTSD when life's various traumas strike.

Many studies have looked at other aspects of victims to understand vulnerability to PTSD. It is important to understand that these studies, though not attempting to blame victims, are all at risk of confounding evidence, of using survey tools which may themselves be flawed, and of measuring characteristics which trauma itself may induce. Among what is reported (12,13,15) are: female gender, lower social class, lower levels of attained education, lower intelligence (as if there is one "intelligence"), neurological "soft signs" (including difference in measured volume of various parts of the brain), homelessness, the presence of pre-extant psychological disturbances, and occurrence of prior traumatic events, including previous sexual assault.

Studies have also examined perpetrators and what they did, as predictors for development of PTSD in their victims. In a provocative study of sexual assault by coaches among elite athletes, Leahy, Pretty, and Tenenbaum (16) hypothesized that the salient factor was not the relationship (parent/parent substitute) or the presence or absence of body violation, but how the perpetrator went about achieving his ends, and what this meant at the time to the victim. In contrast to research mentioned above about victims, most of those they studied were high-achieving, high-performing, previously physically and mentally healthy young people. Quantitatively, Leahy et al. demonstrated an association between the perpetrator being in a position of "trust, authority, and guardianship" and the development of PTSD. Qualitatively, through in-depth interviews with survivors, and separating out a group of those who were subsequently/currently "clinically distressed," they demonstrated that perpetrators whose victims developed PTSD created relationships of powerlessness (victims) and omnipotence (coaches). "What appeared to characterize the experiences of the clinically distressed group was their isolation in a relationship in which the perpetrator successfully controlled the psychological environment. The repeated imposition of the perpetrator's worldview and the lack (due to isolating and silencing strategies) of alternative reference points may result in the victim adopting the perpetrator's viewpoint." This is expressed by a male participant as follows:

> Although at the time, I (pause), I didn't really, uhm (long pause), I suppose I did wonder how he could get an erection uhm (long pause) in front of me, but I didn't even (pause), I didn't really think that he was getting off on it. Uhm (pause), because it was always presented as, uhm (pause), education and that sort of thing.

Leahy et al. pointed out that in their study, as in others, there was a positive correlation between the level of authority and trust and the amount of invasiveness or body penetration involved in the abuse—so that they could not isolate the extent to which the "grooming" of the victim alone had predicted subsequent psychic derangement.

Intimately related to the perpetrator's methods are the victim's feelings and reactions at the time of the abuse. McNally (13), in a review of controversies in the study of PTSD, stresses the "moral complexity" of trauma in people as compared to animal models. "Toxic (levels of) fear" can be induced in animals by threatening their survival, and subsequent lab experiments done to understand a PTSD-like syndrome of avoidance and vigilance which occurs. In his studies of Vietnam veterans, however, he uncovered guilt and shame (at having committed atrocities) as precursors to its development. Shame at being a victim, and accepting blame projected by perpetrators, may be part of why sexual violence has such a strong ability to predict subsequent PTSD, particularly in women but also in men.

Dissociation at the time of trauma seems also to predict subsequent PTSD. (We shall explore more about this state in Chapter 4.) McNally reviewed a number of studies of civilians exposed to motor vehicle trauma and violent crime, and found that "feelings of unreality, time distortion, a sense of bodily distortion" as well as evidence of sympathetic arousal immediately following the event, were all correlated positively. Of course, the severity of the event, as experienced by the person, could be related to how much dissociation was needed to cope with the event, and one cannot tease that out by such retrospective studies.

Finally, interpersonal relations following a trauma are key elements in the path to PTSD. Arata (as quoted in Ullman and Filipas (17)) noted that abuse disclosure to others decreased intrusive and alerting symptoms of PTSD. Ullman studied college students with histories of childhood sexual abuse and showed that the greater extent of disclosure yielded less PTSD regardless of the age at which it occurred. Others, however, have commented on the negative effects many children endure when attempting to disclose as children. Ullman's studies also demonstrated the effect of "negative social reactions" on increasing PTSD symptoms. This is relevant to us as medical providers. Positive reactions included offers of support and belief in the validity of the victim's experience. Negative reactions, in contrast, encompassed attempts to control the teller's decision-making, blame of teller, attaching a stigma to teller (treating them differently afterwards), discouraging talking, or "egocentric" responses (talking about the listener's issues instead of the teller's). Her study emphasized that the positive effects of disclosure are more than outweighed if the listener gives back one or more of these negative responses.

Thinking about disclosure within families or to interested others, we can imagine that if a person undergoing a trauma had grown up with the benefits of a secure attachment with someone, with its attendant benefits of the development of good social discrimination, trust in others, and flexibility, such a person would be more likely to know whom to tell, when, and perhaps to find the right person within one's own family.

As clinicians, we are trained to be skeptical and filtering listeners. We also come with our own histories of attachment—secure, or flawed. Many of us are aware of the controversies surrounding "false memory" syndrome, as well as of the tendency for the human being to try to capitalize on the positive benefits of a negative experience (financial, sympathy, publicity, etc.) What is important to focus on, I believe, is the phrase "belief in the validity of . . ." In a one-on-one encounter in which one person (a patient) is relating a prior experience, we are listening for that person's experience—for what happened to them, and within them—not necessarily for what happened. That is what needs to matter for us.

Screening for PTSD

Being heard can be healing. We can increase the likelihood that we will identify someone with PTSD by being aware that it is "out there." This book exists to raise awareness. There are many other educational resources. A medical encounter, however, has multiple demands placed upon it by patient, provider, and increasingly by government and insurance companies. Hidden symptoms are not so easily brought to the surface. This is especially so when one's patient has suppressed or forgotten their traumas or has reacted to them by avoiding topics which bring it up. In addition, all too frequently our patients have had negative encounters before, either with health care providers or others in a position to "help."

Researchers, therefore, have devised short screening tools which will aid the busy clinician in the recognition of PTSD. These are similar to other questionnaires that exist for other commonly ignored but extremely important conditions such as dementia (the short list), depression (Beck Depression inventory), or alcoholism (the CAGE questions) and others. They are easily administered in the office setting, take a minimum of time, and are reasonably sensitive tests. Of course, their positive predictive value, as in any test administered, depends on the frequency of the condition in the population tested. As a provider, one needs to be adept at identifying clues—epidemiologic, behavioral, symptom-based, verbal—to know which patients need screening and closer scrutiny.

For example, Kimerling et al. (18) reported on the utility and their validation of the Breslau 7-question screen (see box). In their study, the screen was self-administered. Those questions could fairly easily be incorporated into a face-to-face encounter as well, although the seven questions might be difficult to recall for a clinician using them only occasionally. I personally find it easier to keep copies of such screening devices in an accessible file and bring them into an encounter as needed.

Breslau Short Screening Scale for PTSD

In your life, have you ever had any experience that was so frightening, horrible, or upsetting that, in the past month . . .

1. Did you avoid being reminded of this experience by staying away from certain places, people, or activities?
2. Did you lose interest in activities that were once important or enjoyable?
3. Did you begin to feel more isolated or distant from other people?
4. Did you find it hard to have love or affection for other people?
5. Did you begin to feel that there was no point in planning for the future?
6. After this experience were you having more trouble than usual falling asleep or staying asleep?
7. Did you become jumpy or get easily startled by ordinary noises or movements?

Breslau et al. proposed that using a cutoff of four (out of a possible seven) positive answers provided the user with the best discrimination—the best balance of sensitivity and specificity—for that test. In Kimerling's study, waiting-room patients completed the scale in five minutes or so, and their scores were correlated with results of in-depth interviews at a later date. Likelihood of PTSD not surprisingly increased with the score on the test. They also found that the score of 4 provided the best discrimination between those with the disorder and those without, but suggested that, if need be, a provider could scale her efforts to those with the higher scores. They noted that, using interview diagnoses of PTSD as a gold standard, only 38% of those with the disorder had this diagnosis previously noted in their medical chart.

The American Association of Family Practice has published a Point of Care (PC) guideline for PTSD screening on their website. Writing about the guideline, Ebell (19) elaborates on the PC-PTSD screening device, a four-item series now required in the assessment of returning combat veterans. The questions read as follows:

PC-PTSD Screening Instrument

In your life have you ever had any experience that was so frightening, horrible, or upsetting that in the past month you:

- Have had nightmares about it or thought about it when you did not want to?
- Tried hard not to think about it or went out of your way to avoid situations that reminded you of it?
- Were constantly on guard, watchful, or easily startled?
- Felt numb or detached from others, activities, or your surroundings?

A score of 3 or 4 is a positive response.

Finally, Lang and Stein (20) studied characteristics of several screening tools derived from more cumbersome "parents" and demonstrated reasonable validity for even a two-item tool. The two items chosen, from a list of 17 which comprise the PCL-C civilian version, were:

- Do you have intrusive recollections, memories thoughts or images of what happened to you, when you don't mean to be remembering them?
- Are you upset when reminded of what happened to you?

A third item with the best correlation had to do with whether the person felt hyper alert or overly vigilant. They recognized the need for time efficiency in primary care, and they found the two questions correlated reasonably with the longer, 17-item research tool.

Ultimately, the utility of such screening devices will be proven or disproven in practice. Most often cues and clues in the patient's words, or fragments of their experience or behavior, might be what leads us to suspect PTSD, and then perhaps pursue a path (including the above screens) which may validate or invalidate its presence. Again, I would emphasize many people have grown up with trauma as a norm. They would not characterize what happened to them as "frightening, horrible, or upsetting," and for some of them, it WAS so frightening or horrible that they have completely forgotten it. For such people, an encounter with a doctor who wonders out loud with the patient may startlingly revise their vision of their past.

PTSD and Health Care

PTSD often coexists with other mental disorders. It is associated with anxiety disorders, depression, phobias, and addiction. Often substance abuse is itself linked with trauma. For instance, childhood sexual abuse is more frequent in families where parents are abusing alcohol and drugs. Combat veterans may learn to cope with the stress of battle by availing themselves of readily available addicting drugs, cigarettes, and alcohol. Under such circumstances, victims may come to addiction either by repeated exposure or genetic predisposition. It is important to remember that people can be addicted not just to drugs but to such things as food and work, the immersion in which can have temporary soothing, anxiety-relieving qualities. The effects of addiction, the effects of addictive substances, and the symptoms of depression may all prompt repeated medical encounters.

PTSD causes increased visits to health care settings. Kartha et al. (21) presented data derived from a study of English-speaking primary care patients at an urban "safety-net" hospital. Eighty-one percent of those approached agreed to participate. Of the 592 patients who did so, 80% had had at least one traumatic exposure, and 22% were found to have PTSD at the time of the study, which lasted a mean of 11.9 years. Subjects with PTSD had over twice the number of hospitalizations and mental health visits than those without it, though (in contrast to other studies) they did not visit primary care settings more often. Subjects with a history of trauma alone, without PTSD, did not have these findings. The surprising finding regarding primary care, the authors felt, might have been influenced by a high baseline use of primary care in their entire subject population—that is, by selection criteria for their study.

Stein et al. (22) studied English-speaking outpatients at a university-affiliated primary care setting staffed by family practitioners. This was a different group. Only 48% of those approached agreed to participate. Sixty-six percent of participants had had at least one traumatic exposure, most commonly being a witness to serious injury/death (34%) or sexual victimization (23%). PTSD prevalence was 11.8% by their definitions. The group with PTSD was much more likely to have been medically hospitalized in the past six months (16.7% vs. 1.4%), to have visited an emergency room in that period of time (44% vs. 12%), or to have utilized any medical provider more than six times (44% vs. 24%) in the past six months.

Finally, Walker et al. (23) studied the effects of PTSD on health care costs using a mailed questionnaire, with subsequent interview validation, of a sample of 1,225 women enrollees in an HMO in 1996–97. This was a staff model health maintenance organization, where costs were closely tracked, ER and specialty visits discouraged by the structure of the HMO itself, and hospitalization minimalized and monitored. Twenty-five percent of those completing the questionnaire in this majority white, middle-class sample had a history of childhood sexual abuse. Ten percent of all the sample (not just those with prior abuse) had PTSD. Using the PCL, a well-validated, research-oriented PTSD tool, the entire group was categorized as having low, moderate, or high PTSD scores. Adjusting for concomitant chronic diseases and depression scores, the high PTSD scorers had twice the health care costs as the lowest. These higher scores were not for mental health costs or hospitalization, but mostly for primary care and pharmacy. Adjusting out the factors of chronic disease and depression may underestimate the stress that PTSD places on the health care system, since it is often associated with both. And, as the authors pointed out, in systems where the "gateways" to hospitalization are less well controlled than theirs, the gap could have been higher for that entity as well, as it was in Stein's study.

People with PTSD may find their way into the health care system for many reasons associated with but not explained only by the disorder itself. Most do not present with anxiety symptoms per se. They may come for help with addictions, with the burdens of substance abuse, bothered by depressive symptoms, or, as the above studies suggest implicitly, for help with bodily complaints. They may, or may not, have more body-based illnesses. But they also somatize. They express and experience their distress in their bodies, without linking it with emotional distress or without being able to connect it emotionally to old, distressing experiences. Disorders of pain, gastrointestinal function, sleep, muscle function, and sexual function, to name a few, frequently appear in this category. One of the clinician's greatest challenges is to distinguish the "functional" disorder from the "organic" in such a situation. Another is to know when the sufferer of functional illness HAS an organic disease. As the old saying goes, "even a hypochondriac has to die some time." But perhaps the biggest challenge of all is to find a way to HELP the sufferer of a functional illness.

For one thing, it often seems that the practitioner and patient are speaking two different languages. The doctor may have decided as well as she can that this illness is functional, or "not real." The patient knows this, has various reactions to that knowledge, and most of all knows that they "still have that pain." It appears that many traditional medical approaches to functional illnesses are of limited utility, so that the doctor may feel helpless, impotent, or bored. That patient can easily become frustrated and discouraged. There appears to be an impasse.

Underlying this deadlock may be the nature of trauma itself, and how it affects the language function of human beings. Sexual trauma in particular often occurs under the cloak of shame and secrecy, perpetuated by frightening threats by the perpetrator on the victim not to tell anyone lest something even more dreadful happen. The adult survivor may experience terror, amnesia, and shame at sharing *any* closely held memory—not just memories of the incident(s) themselves.

More fundamentally, the survivor of trauma often believes that he will not be believed if he attempts to tell what happened. All too often, this is actually the case. Even if a victim has never tried to tell others, however, sexual, criminal, and war crimes often violate our normal codes of conduct and beliefs about the right ordering of life. Victims who understand this will know they are on dangerous ground if they try to tell.

Finally, as Primo Levi has discussed, there is something in the nature of trauma that defies the use of language as a tool. It is as if words themselves mock the would-be teller. A survivor hears herself speak, knowing that no word, or combination of words, can convey the intensity or complexity of actions and feelings involved in some acts of abuse. For this kind of communication, perhaps only the nonverbal suffices. That kind of communication we receive in art (movies, plays, music, painting, metaphor). That kind of communication can also, however, be conveyed by the suffering and actions of a human body. Both disease and actions arising in response to feelings in this context may be understood as information about PTSD, about a story of prior abuse or neglect. And in this context, our own feelings and reactions may help to tell the story as well.

Characteristic Behaviors Stemming from PTSD

Implicit in the *DSM 5* definition of post-traumatic stress disorder are some common characteristics of people who have it. People with PTSD have trouble with "boundaries." Strong intrusive experiences and reactions to them lead sufferers to intrude on others with their anxieties and concerns. Their fears and experiences lead them not to follow the normal rules of engagement—patient waiting, modulated expression, and so on. They may sexualize or make violent their secular relationships (with spouses, friends, and caregivers.) They are prone to re-traumatization by aspects of events which most people can tune out—for instance, invasive medical procedures. They, or their behaviors, demand special attention. The attention they get is often not what they hoped for or need.

The avoidance phenomena of PTSD also deserve mention here. People with PTSD may promise to carry out a task (e.g., make an appointment for a colonoscopy) but fail to be able to do so. When asked why, they often have no cogent explanation "I just never got to it" or "I couldn't bring myself to do it." On the other hand, when they finally do come to do it, they may insist on general anesthesia. They may appear remarkably unattached—to the office, the provider, or sometimes to anyone. They may have unusually fatalistic responses to encouragement to care for themselves, being unable to partner with the doctor in successfully managing a chronic illness over time, for instance. These people are easy to ignore and hard to understand.

Some of the threads of this discussion are re-created in the case of Elora. The momentum and features of her organic illness created intensity enough. Not knowing her, and her issues, made life more difficult for her doctors and her as we navigated through its demands. Her own life story, unknown to us at the onset and unprocessed by her, constituted the third arm of a "triple threat." This patient's illness challenged everyone's resilience.

Elora

Elora first presented years ago to a young colleague who was just beginning in practice. This doctor particularly enjoyed caring for young women and their problems. The patient was 39 and the mother of three young children. All she wanted was a referral to her old obstetrician for a tubal ligation. "She smokes 2.5 packs of cigarettes per week. She has occasional alcohol. She denies any sexual activity and does not use any contraception because of that. She states that her diet is good in calcium. Pt. did not want to divulge any further information. Pt. refused exam at this time . . . She states that she will come back after she gets to know me better to get the rest of this done. . . ." Between the lines, we hear wariness on the part of the patient, and some frustration on the part of the doctor. Was there any conversation about the patient's reluctance, where it was coming from? Was the paradox of "coming back after getting to know me better" explored? We do not know these things.

In addition, the patient had control of the situation. She had picked out her procedure, her specialist, and she just wanted the rubber stamp to go ahead—which, later that year, she did.

One year later, Elora returned to our clinic. Her first doctor had moved away and now I would be seeing her. She was a striking, fit woman with tight fitting clothes, dyed blonde hair, and a tough attitude. Her right arm had been in pain, and tingling, for several days. This had begun out of the blue. She had been told in the past that she had Raynaud's syndrome. This was different than in the past, she said. Her hand felt cold, all the time, and ached enough that she was uncomfortable a good deal of the day. Her hand did not change color. Her examination showed cool, but normal-colored hands, right more than left; soft tissue tenderness at the radial portion of the wrist. I could palpate a brachial but not radial pulse on the right. Passive and active range of motion were ok. There were no carpal tunnel findings. She denied use of oral contraceptives.

I remember feeling concerned, puzzled. I remember sensing her fear and her native intelligence. I felt as if a wild animal had come into the clinic, someone who didn't want to be there, who would only use me as a last resort but who had run out of home remedies and was worried she was running out of time. Her anxiety and her unanswerable questions propelled me to immediate action.

I told Elora about her lack of radial pulse, and that this was going to be "something weird," and to be prepared for that. Patients understandably want us to know what to do, and how to do it. They, and we, don't like to say, "I have no idea what this is." But it's better, I think, to share the not-knowing together than to pretend we do know and send the patient out on a wild goose chase. In this case, I conveyed my allegiance and ignorance, and she ended up on a wild goose chase anyway.

I got her an appointment that day with a vascular surgeon. The person she saw was not my first choice, but everyone else was in the OR or working elsewhere. This surgeon was someone who dislikes being interrupted for "trivial" complaints, even if patients or primary caregivers are worried. At the same time, he gets anxious when problems are major and require his intervention. Every good doctor feels that way: it is healthy "clinical anxiety." His anxiety is at times projected onto the patient, or the referring physician, who then appears to him as a colossal pain. I regarded him as a difficult person with whom to work, and someone whom I experienced as demeaning to me at times. He is a competent surgeon.

"This 40-year-old patient is referred today acutely for complaints of right arm pain and 'lack of pulses' in her right arm." This surgeon found Elora's fingertips cooler bilaterally, palpable pulses (all of them) in both arms, and normal dopplers. She had focal tenderness over the wrist. "I don't really have a dx for the patient at this point in time, although I do not think that this is any kind of clear-cut vasospastic disorder or manifestation of any type of acute thrombosis." He thought that she perhaps had tendonitis, referred her to a hand surgeon, gave her anti-inflammatories, and ice. Elora did not want to see him again, disappointed and angered by the lack of clarity. The surgeon then made an appointment for two months for Elora to see Dr. F, the man I'd originally wanted her to see.

Six days later Elora saw the hand surgeon. I did not hear from him but called the patient before I left on vacation for two weeks. According to Elora he agreed that she had a tendonitis and prescribed a new anti-inflammatory. She had tried that, and others, without relief—even if she took them all at the same time! I gave her a small dose of a narcotic and called the hand surgeon's office with my concerns. They booked an MRI.

I then went on vacation.

One week later, Elora called my office. Note from the secretary: "Patient quite upset and wants to speak with doc re MRI results—Dr. R (the hand surgeon) on vacation . . . (good luck with this one) (not a nice patient)." A second encouragement: "I'm afraid if you don't call her she'll just show up and cause a big scene." My colleague, a new provider with a soft-spoken, matter-of-fact style, "spoke with patient—discussed MRI with patient (increased fluid in soft tissues), instructed to keep appointment with Dr. R."

One week later I was still on vacation, and Elora called my partner again. The receptionist gave the doctor another note: "has an appointment with (hand surgeon) . . . but wants to be seen today. She can't take the pain. She wouldn't let me say anything just kept screaming." (last two words highlighted by receptionist). My partner arranged for her to be seen the next day by the hand surgeon and noted "patient is very belligerent."

There are no further notes on the chain of events, but I believe the hand surgeon, after seeing her, sent her for repeat arterial upper extremity dopplers. These were carried out a week or so later. They now showed "moderate occlusive arterial disease in the right upper extremity," without evidence on maneuvers for thoracic outlet syndrome. There appeared to be a stenotic area near the brachial artery, and possibly an aneurysm in the subclavian on the right. The patient then met with Dr. F, and an arteriogram was arranged for one week later.

Was progress being made? The group of doctors were feeling their way to a diagnosis in the face of shifting signals, contradictory information, and pictures which couldn't tell all. At the same time, a personal story was unfolding. Elora was someone who "wouldn't take no for an answer"; who "wouldn't listen . . . would just keep screaming." There was a primal quality to her, a fierce sticking up for herself but also a kind of inability to elaborate in words on pain and need. Closer to a diagnosis, she didn't hesitate, either, to fire someone by whom she felt wronged, even if they could help her, even if it was clear she needed their skills. There was a fierce loyalty to herself and her pride which overrode any constraints to behave rationally, civilly, or arguably in her own best interest. There was also a black and white quality to her judgments. If the first vascular surgeon became despised, she was looking for another who would become a rescuer, someone who could do no wrong.

One month into "knowing" Elora, then, we should have begun to wonder about complex post-traumatic stress disorder. Why? Certainly, we knew little about her previous life or its difficulties. We didn't know anything about intrusive or avoidant symptoms. The physical problems she was having were provoking fear and agitated behavior, perhaps on a continuum with anyone suffering from a progressive undiagnosed, painful disorder. But she seemed, at least to the front desk staff, to be someone who was uninterested or unable to "regulate affect" ("not a nice person"); she was unfazed by her own belligerence and aware of its potential power in the short term to garner attention; trust emerged as a MAJOR issue; and underneath all was the worry about being properly cared for.

I, meanwhile, was struggling to catch up after my vacation.

Two days after her arteriogram Elora's arm turned "blue," and she called Dr. F. He met her in the emergency department and became her hero. At this point her exam revealed a "cool, blanched" right arm without palpable pulses. There was a palpable subclavian artery aneurysm and "fullness" in the supraclavicular area. Angiography was again done and showed bilateral cervical ribs, the subclavian artery aneurysm, believed to be caused by the compression of the cervical rib on the right, and a new embolus to the brachial artery. Elora was admitted to the hospital, and lytic therapy was tried and failed. So, the next day, she was taken to the operating room for a brachial embolectomy. She was temporarily anticoagulated. The following day, after reversal, she returned to the OR for a right cervical rib resection, aneurysm resection, and a short, technically difficult graft to the subclavian artery. Following these maneuvers, her hand warmed up and an ulnar pulse was palpable. She had an uneventful postoperative course. She left the hospital four days after the second surgery. I visited her. She was intensely relieved.

I saw Elora three days after discharge at her request. She was taking almost no narcotics, as she disliked the effect on her thinking. After washing floors, doing laundry, and actively caring for her three children, her two incisions seemed more swollen, and she was worried. She applied ice with improvement, but she came in to have the area checked. She was exquisitely dressed, and her incisions were also healing beautifully. A good brachial and a minimal radial artery were now palpable.

Four days later, she saw Dr. F. He found all healing well. He noted that she was getting an aneurysm of the other side (left subclavian) upon review of the initial angiogram, and would need elective left cervical rib resection. Two weeks later, healing had progressed further, and the third surgery was planned.

Two months after the original surgery, however, she developed increased finger numbness on the right, and saw Dr. F. He felt her graft was nonfunctional. The right hand was cool, no pulses palpable. She was taken that day to the operating room, where it appeared her first rib was compressing the graft, so it was also resected, along with a thrombectomy in the graft area. That evening and the next day, she complained of chest pain. I saw her the morning after surgery, and I recall not making sense of her pain nor of any findings in her chest. A kind of inability to think diagnostically fuzzed my head. The surgical house staff, who had seen her earlier, also could not make sense of her symptoms and had moved on to their considerable workload for the day. Over the course of the morning, she became increasingly insistent and belligerent with the nurses. A chest x-ray finally done revealed a large whiteout of the right chest, and she again lost arm pulses. She was promptly returned to the OR, where a large hemothorax (from the first rib resection), as well as a recurrent clot in the subclavian graft, were both appreciated. Her hematocrit dropped to 19. An intraoperative chest tube was placed, and a new carotid to axillary bypass graft was created with saphenous vein harvested from her right leg. The surgeons had tried to work with the original graft, but "dense adhesions" around the original anastomosis made it impossible. Postoperatively, she slowly improved. Her arm was again well-perfused. Her chest tube was eventually removed, though she left the hospital still with fluid and blood in her pleural cavity. This also gradually resorbed.

I feel to this day that I failed Elora that post-op morning. I say this not to beat my breast, but to remark that I, too, like the first vascular surgeon, couldn't "hear" (in the sense of being disturbed enough by) her symptoms. I am not a surgeon and can't fix surgical problems. But I can and usually do have intuitions with patients; that morning, my intuition was dulled. The tiger had roared into a void.

I do not know if having formally "named" her PTSD would have helped me or her other doctors. It might have. When interpersonal trauma is occurring to a child, there are generally four actors in the scenario: the victim, the perpetrator, the person who might have/could have protected the patient (or perhaps could not), and the bystanders, the rest of society, who probably have intimations of what is happening but are too frightened/uninvolved/disbelieving to act. Often, when dealing with a patient with PTSD, we will see these characters re-emerge, with the actors changing roles without notice. Elora, for instance, had already been both victim (patient with disease), perpetrator (battering my front desk), and rescuer (firing her first surgeon). Dr. F and I had been rescuers; but now, both the surgeons and I were the dumbstruck bystanders, being given clues but failing to register or act on them. Had I run through this checklist that morning, would I have seen what I was doing?

The patient slowly healed—again. She had an uneventful post-op visit with Dr. F. She called me about a sore throat but refused to come to see me.

Two months after her third surgery, however, she came in for her first "new patient physical exam" with me. Our practice prefers to do these initially on new patients BEFORE something like the events above occur, partly to foster a working relationship in case of disasters such as these. Really, we had been working in the dark, Elora and I.

"Since (her third operation) she has been disabled. She has been home with her husband whom she does not like, whom she finds verbally abusive." It had been upsetting not to be able to get out and work, but she didn't feel she was depressed. "She wants to get the (final) operation over with so that she can enjoy her summer, return to work and seek some independence."

This was the first time the abuse word was spoken. Elora's experience was that she was living with it, out of necessity, in order to raise her children.

She had been born and brought up locally, one of three. She had attended high school but married partway through, then divorced at 22. She then married again at 31, having three children with this husband in four years. Since her kids had arrived, she had held down two part-time jobs, one doing manual labor for her town and another in a local supermarket. She had quit smoking after her first operation this past year, occasionally however "sneaking a cigarette from her husband." She kept in shape over the years doing martial arts, until this past September. She had breastfed all of her children—her only daughter for the longest, over a year. All three pregnancies were uneventful; she reported one miscarriage. She had had several syncopal episodes which she attributed to low blood sugar, as they occurred when she had been fasting.

Physically, she finally had a clear chest, well-healed scars, a warmer right hand, still cooler than the left, and some umbilical jewelry. I felt she could undergo her final surgery. One month later, she had an elective left cervical rib resection. She had some neurogenic pain and numbness which was significant postoperatively, thought to be due to intraoperative traction on her brachial plexus. She went home three days following the procedure, with gradual improvement in the brachial plexus symptoms.

I saw her a month later. She was worried only about a bump on the back of her tongue. She appeared to have just an inflamed posterior papilla, knowledge of which relieved her greatly.

Four months later, she called complaining of left arm tingling; the arm felt dead transiently, then recovered. She came in that same evening. If she lay on her back, her arms would tingle and feel numb, then recover as she got up and got walking. Overall, she felt she was improving. She had a new sexual partner (not her husband). She was remembering getting transfused; wanted an HIV test. On exam, her arms and hands and pulses were at her new baseline, and perfusion looked excellent. Her pelvic exam was normal. An HIV test was negative.

The underlying themes, as she returned to health, were her bodily integrity; sexual health; increasing unhappiness with her husband; truthfulness and trusting; self-preservation. Two years into our relationship, with all our ups and downs, Elora was "coming back after getting to know me better." In addition, she was sharing concerns about private matters. Was she normal? Was sexual activity ok? Did she dare look outside of a marriage which felt abusive, for comfort and love?

Over the next couple of years, she was seen for a variety of self-limited problems. Eventually, she had another general exam. The previous summer had been good—she'd spent time at the beach, at an amusement park with her kids, and was involved with one of her son's sports. She was trying to change careers, studying computers. If she spent more than two hours on the keyboard, she felt numb and stiff in several fingers of the right hand. She had quit her city job. "She finds that if she takes one mg of clonazepam daily she feels much better." She takes it to this day. Her wounds were healed, her left subclavian aneurysm was possibly palpable, and she had blood in her stool for unclear reasons. Detailed GI review of systems revealed nothing. "Elora became acutely agitated at hearing this" (the guaiac positive stool), "burst into tears and could not allow a strange person to draw her blood, and generally told me that this was going to be a 'two Klonepin day.'" A noninvasive workup initially revealed more occult blood on subsequent stools, and I advised a workup one week later. She again became tearful, telling me "I want to be done with hospitals." She did not want to return to the local hospital where so much had happened, right now. I referred her elsewhere, and she did endoscopies promptly. Colonoscopy was negative, and a GI series revealed duodenitis.

She returned a month after the tests to discuss them. "Elora tells me now that she frequently has mid epigastric pain after 'yelling,' i.e., during arguments with her husband, and describes a recent one that she had. This has been true of her since she was a young child. She also drinks a six pack at a time at night on some weekends, though not much during the week." (Four months later, Elora read her own chart while waiting for me in an exam room and corrected the last sentence. She often split a six pack with her sister each weekend night.) I treated her with Ranitidine.

She returned at the end of that year. Ranitidine had improved the argument-associated pain. We decided to stop it. Something, however, had changed. "Patient provided additional social history. She was raised in a violent home by a father who physically abused her mother, her, and her older sister. (The patient) describes herself as the one who would defiantly refuse to cry in the face of her father's blows. Her older sister (on the other hand) would start to cry before they even started. Consequently, Elora was beaten more severely." When the patient was eight years old, their mother took her and her sister out of the house and left the father. They had to live in the projects. Patient at 11 moved out of her home and moved in with her grandmother and went to high school until the age of 16. She then married for the first time for about six years. Her husband was in the Air Force, and she did complete high school near the base where they lived. At 21, they separated, having developed different interests and having had no children. She then lived on her own for about 12 years before marrying the man with whom she had her family, whom she was with when I met her.

"She is amazed that her mother would let go of her. She states that her mother was very depressed and spent much of her (the patient's) high school years in bed. She can't imagine letting any of her children leave her household, the way she was allowed to go."

So, there it is, the skeletal outline of an abusive past. Elora's mother, after orchestrating an escape into safety (and poverty) for her brood, falls into a deep depression, leaving Elora to fend for herself. By age eight, Elora had learned defiance, denial of pain, self-reliance, an aggressive stance against someone twice her size. By 11, she had also chosen independence over what her mother could give her. By 16, she had married her high school sweetheart, at 21 divorced, and after years of independence, she chose marriage to a man who proved to be violent. She had also learned martial arts; she was physically very strong; she had mastered the art of her own attractiveness and what it could get for her. She had never learned the nuances of her own needs; she had rarely been listened to. It was hard for her to tell the difference between normal and abnormal in her body, and consequently she was prey to enormous anxiety about it. Finally, it was almost impossible for her to be impaired and in need, to be vulnerable; she had built her life around being invincible. Maybe that was why "she wouldn't let me say anything, she just kept screaming."

Over the next couple of years, Elora tried and could not return to her old job—the loads on her arms were too much for her impaired circulation. She found a new job as a hostess. She wondered if I would serve as a reference for her (I said I couldn't). Her menstrual cycle became at times irregular, and she wondered about menopause. Irregular bleeding at times made her very worried. She lived with ongoing symptoms with her arms—especially while sleeping. She kept in yearly touch with the surgeon. She saw her children through latency and adolescent years. During her annual exams, she allowed pelvic exams but refused rectal exams, perhaps recalling the trouble I had found earlier and the sharing that had ensued. Over the years, her husband moved to the couch, then out of the house entirely, though she worried about keeping her household together without him. She repeatedly denied that he was physically abusive, "just" verbally so.

At her last annual exam, I wrote, "Since she last had a physical, (Elora) separated from her husband, who is now living with his sister. He is trying to get more (time with children), he is trying to take away the house, they are going to court soon, and her oldest son has been foulmouthed towards her. She and her son were in a physical struggle after her son pushed her after she fell on him, and she eventually broke a choke hold by biting him, and the son a week later reported the incident to the school nurse, which brought the Department of Children and Families in. After a morning of investigation, they have left her alone." Her daughter was close to her, worried about losing her, overweight. Elora continued to work as a hostess. She was still having regular menses. She occasionally saw an old boyfriend. She had some forearm tenderness during work at times. She worried about a clot. Her exam was normal.

PTSD and Elora

Elora's childhood experiences with threats to her well-being were unknown to all of us at the time she presented with her major illness. We barely knew her. She had rebuffed standard initial attempts. I present her case in detail not because "PTSD was the problem" but because aspects of it, if not met and dealt with, threatened to undermine medical care of her serious current problems. The vagaries of her case and the seriousness of it illustrate the importance of being knowledgeable about and equipped to deal with the anxiety, memory, and behavioral sequelae of trauma.

Elora had organic disease. She had cervical ribs, true thoracic outlet syndrome, brachial aneurysms, clot, acute and chronic arterial insufficiency, and GI distress. How much all of this related to repeated beatings during her latency years we cannot know. Some of its manifesting in early mid-life was related to her jobs, which involved heavy lifting and moving. Her schooling, limited by circumstances directly linked to her violent upbringing, failed to prepare her to do a lot else, though she clearly possesses the intelligence to do so. She finished high school by dint of her own perseverance. Additionally, she had dealt with past threats by working out and becoming physically strong. We can wonder if her upper body musculature contributed to the crowding in her thoracic outlet. Clearly, she was born with the anatomic substrate for thoracic outlet syndrome, as well.

Elora also brought with her some of the many burdens of a child of trauma. She avoided standard intimacy creation, the primary care relationship. (Perhaps it wasn't the right person.) Intimations of "something wrong" sowed panic in her. (People without a trauma history might have panicked as well at some of what Elora experienced.) Violence became associated with every generation of men in her life, and she seemed bemused, if not unknowing, about this. Having not yet processed or worked out her early violent past, she lived it repeatedly.

If we didn't know that she had had a violent childhood, we could have guessed. Elora battered the front desk with her needs. She complained bitterly about and verbally despised the first surgeon, who told me later, "I'm not going to let my reputation be ruined by some little twit." Her illness pursued an abrupt and choppy, chaotic course.

Guidelines: Caring for Persons with PTSD

How might we care for someone with PTSD, after listening to Elora's case?

- PTSD is "real," and it belongs on the problem list along with everything else. It demands "management."
- When unmanaged, caregivers of a patient with it become actively involved in a trauma drama as perpetrators, victims, "should-have-knowns," or foolish or wanton bystanders, singly or in shifting combinations. (see Chapter 5). The primary caregiver—not the patient, and certainly not those who know the patient less well—must do the managing. This includes self-management. On the day of her chest bleed, all of Elora's doctors, including myself, were ignorant bystanders for a few precious hours. Her first surgeon shifted between victim and perpetrator—as did Elora herself. Our office staff felt abused and powerless to do much besides describe and complain about the patient's behavior.
- Management involves, first and foremost, a profound respect for the patient. We have to believe in the truth of the patient's symptoms. This is not

the same as believing everything the patient says is "true." It means that there is a story worth exploring in what the patient says. It is also not to be expected that the listener will understand what the truth is right away, or even after repeated telling. Some things may take years to understand. Some will defy understanding.

- Management also involves respect for the coping strategies, the altered memories, and the sheer survival of the patient against adversity. It must also hold out the hope that the patient's coping and style of living can broaden and get healthier, over time and in the context of a relationship consisting of care and concern, boundaries around behavior, and focused on the safety, learning, and well-being of the patient as well as the caregiver and health care system.
- The body has speech of its own for everyone, but particularly for those who grew up with trauma. The body's symptoms, and its involvement in the behavior of its owner, have much to say to the patient and prepared listener. The medical practitioner must be prepared to be the first to hear and to attempt to understand. The patient may not want or need to be able to know for a while. There must also be preparation of both parties NOT to understand at first, and for a long while. This takes a lot of trust on the part of the patient and honesty on the part of the practitioner.
- Guidelines for everyone's behavior—the provider, the patient, the assisting staff—are essential, and deviations from those guidelines are important clues that something is or has gone on. Rules about being intruded upon, yelled at, taken advantage of, or approached sexually provide a sort of "platform" upon which we as providers, and our staff, can stand. "We can't do our job as it needs to be done when we (you/me) are engaged in this sort of behavior. And we want to do our job right. And you hired me to do my job right." "We have run out of time today, but let's plan on another visit soon." "You don't need to yell at me, I am not your (father, abuser, whoever)." "I hear what you are saying, and I am sorry I can't respond in the way you say you want right now."
- Proper management includes choosing the right consultants and settings for specialty care and educating those people on the needs of your patient. The better you know your consulting staff and the healthier your relationship with them, the better you can prepare them to bring their best selves to your patient. Those on the "front lines" bear the brunt of the kind of "assault" with which a past trauma propels a patient to begin a relationship; we need to process it with our patients and within ourselves as best we can, before helping to integrate the patient into a system of care.

- It is the primary provider's job to do "psycho-education" with a patient with PTSD. "Repetitive, negative experiences happen to many people who have suffered what you have." "You have an interesting symptom for which I have no explanation." "We are working on a problem that is going to require a lot of patience." "I don't feel that I know you very well, but I would be interested in knowing more about that."
- Don't expect it to go away. Do expect the development of trust to be slow and rocky.

Don't underestimate the tools we all have of respect and listening. Remember, this person (with PTSD) was once a small child, with the same needs as yours or your children's. What happened to them lives in the realm of your "worst fears" for those you love—including your own family, and yourself.

References

1. Oliver M, "This Morning Again in the Dusty Pines," *New and Selected Poems*, Beacon Press, 1992. Reprinted by the permission of The Charlotte Sheedy Literary Agency as agent for the author. Copyright © 1992 by Mary Oliver with permission of Bill Reichblum.
2. PTSD formally entered the nosology of psychiatric disorders in 1980, when it was included in the *DSM III*, largely at the behest of Vietnam veterans who were personally familiar with the disorder. It has most likely been around since the beginning of time. It is related to "hysteria" suffered by Victorian women, to WWI veterans' "shell-shock," and so on, 2022.
3. Reprinted with permission from the *Diagnostic and Statistical Manual of Mental Disorders, Fifth Edition*, Text Revision (Copyright © 2022). American Psychiatric Association. All Rights Reserved, 2022.
4. Herman, Cloitre, and Ford, 2009, as cited in Courtois C, and Ford J, *Treatment of Complex Trauma A Sequenced, Relationship-Based Approach*, pp. 47–48. Guilford Press, 2013.
5. Briere J, Scott C, and Jones J, "The effects of trauma," in Briere, J., and Scott, C. (eds.) *Principles of Trauma Therapy, A Guide to Symptoms, Evaluation, and Treatment*, Sage Publications, Inc, 2015.
6. See, for instance, any of Allan Schore's comprehensive books integrating basic science and clinical work, e.g., *The Science of the Art of Psychotherapy*, WW Norton, 2012.
7. Nemeroff C, "Neurobiological consequences of childhood trauma," *Journal of Clinical Psychiatry* 65(suppl 1): 18–28, 2004.
8. Lanius R, Lanius U, Fisher J, and Ogden P, "Psychological Trauma and the Brain: Toward a Neurobiological Treatment Model," in Ogden, P, Minton, K, and Pain, C (eds.) *Trauma and the Body, A Sensorimotor Approach to Psychotherapy*, pp. 139–161. WW Norton, 2006.
9. Liverzon I, Britton JC, and Phan KI, "Neural correlates of traumatic recall in post- traumatic stress disorder," *Stress* 6(3): 151–156, 2003.
10. Bremner JD, "Effects of traumatic stress on brain structure and function: Relevance to early responses to trauma," *Journal of Trauma & Dissociation* 6(2): 51–68, 2005.
11. Schore A, *Affect Regulation and the Repair of the Self*, WW Norton, 2003.
12. Butterfield M and Becker M, "Posttraumatic stress disorder in women, assessment and treatment in primary care," *Primary Care: Clinics in Office Practice* 29(1): 151–169, 2002.

13. McNally R, "Progress and controversy in the study of posttraumatic stress disorder," *Annual Review of Psychology* 54: 229–252, 2003.
14. Bowlby J, *Attachment and Loss* Vol. I, *Attachment*, 2nd edition, Basic Books, 1982.
15. Scott K, Wolfe D, and Wekerle C, "Maltreatment and trauma: tracking the connections in adolescence," *Child and Adolescent Psychiatric Clinics of North America* 12: 211–230, 2003.
16. Leahy T, Pretty G, and Tenenbaum G, "Perpetrator methodology as predictor of traumatic symptomatology in adult survivors of childhood sexual abuse," *Journal of Interpersonal Violence* 19(5): 521–540, 2004.
17. Ullman S and Filipas H, "Gender differences in social reactions to abuse disclosures, post-abuse coping, and PTSD of child sexual abuse survivors," *Child Abuse and Neglect* 29: 767–782, 2005.
18. Kimerling R, Ouimette P, Prins, A, Nisco P, Lawler C, Cronkite R, Moos, R, "Utility of a short screening scale for DSM-IV PTSD in primary care," *Journal of General Internal Medicine* 21(1): 65–67, 2006.
19. Ebell M, "Screening instruments for post-traumatic stress disorder," *American Family Physician*, www.afp.org/afp, 2007.
20. Lang A and Stein M, "An abbreviated PTSD checklist for use as a screening instrument in primary care," *Behavior Research and Therapy* 43(5): 585–594, 2005.
21. Kartha A, Brower V, Saitz R, Samet J, Keane T, and Liebschutz J, "The impact of trauma exposure and post-traumatic stress disorder on healthcare utilization among primary care patients," *Medical Care* 46 (4): 388–393, 2008.
22. Stein M, McQuaid J, Pedrelli P, Lenox R, and McCahill M, "Posttraumatic stress disorder in the primary care medical setting," *General Hospital Psychiatry* 22(4): 261–269, 2000.
23. Walker E, Katon W, Russo J, Ciechanowski P, Newman E, and Wagner A, "Health care costs associated with posttraumatic stress disorder symptoms in women," *Archives of General Psychiatry* 60: 369–374, 2003.

4
Dissociation

It's a blank, safe, quiet space where Nothing (as opposed to Something—something that feels like overwhelming intrusion associated with pain and other feelings too big to feel, for which you have no words, no responses, no strategies, no guide, no path, no strength, no cunning, just such weakness—no, nothing—just clearly, clearly, best not to go there) happens. At first, it is a whitewashed colorless version of Heaven, but after a while, it's just boring, safe, and seemingly necessary (1).

Introduction

It is nearly impossible to understand the inner world of a traumatized person without some grasp of the concept of dissociation. Dissociation is a defense mechanism commonly encountered in a person coping with a traumatic event or events. It often occurs in an individual during an actual trauma. Equally often, however, it appears long after the event, when external threats stir up memories or feelings associated with the trauma. A medical encounter—with its undertones of inquiry, vulnerability, its concerns about injury, illness, death, and certainly with its likelihood of bodily exposure and intrusion—can certainly be such a threat.

It needs to be said that not all dissociation connotes trauma. Most people dissociate every day—for instance, to deal with boredom during a long drive, to get through a stressful or meaningless meeting, or while watching over children happily at play. One "goes somewhere," then realizes, "I can't account for the last seconds or minutes—I mentally escaped!"

Dissociation linked to trauma can be understood very simply as a "mental escape," but its workings are varied and complex, not simple at all. We shall see that once the clinician enters into a healing relationship with a patient bearing a history of trauma violation, we will be faced with dissociation as well.

Understanding Dissociation as a Defense Mechanism, and More

Just as we know that people are much more than their various diagnoses, past trauma and present dissociation will be but one facet of their personality. They will bring to their relationship with us their strengths and weaknesses, and their characteristic ways of dealing with stress and threat, only one of which will be dissociation. However, dissociation is such a **common** way of dealing with prior abuse that we need to become adept at recognizing it, to avoid it mystifying us and causing **us** to dissociate unwittingly.

The relationship between dissociation and prior trauma is not unlike that between denial and substance abuse. It is often very difficult for the substance abuser to see the extent to which they are being crippled by their addiction. "I only have a few drinks each night." "I only drink beer." "I smoke, but I never inhale." Denial comes hand in hand with the addiction process. In addition, the addicted patient's denial extends to others around her. Family and friends may deny the existence of addiction, excusing the person's behavior or finding "reasons" to overlook it. Co-workers learn to "pretend" it isn't there, rather than confronting it. Think about patients you have had where alcoholism has hidden its face for months or years, despite well-documented signs. The disease progresses, and becomes harder to treat, while everyone is looking away.

So, too, dissociation is likely to accompany our patients' trauma stories and becomes part of their modus operandum. Traumatized patients dissociate when they feel threatened. The threat may be experienced by them as coming from us, from an inquiry, from the prospect or actuality of an examination, or from their own memories or stored pain, completely apart from us. If we don't learn to understand the phenomenon of dissociation, how and why it occurs, we will fail to understand how our patients sense us—and at least as importantly, we won't take in its clues about their history.

Dissociation is a mental process geared toward survival, in which connections between mental representations and experiences are severed. This ligation disables a person's ability to experience all aspects of a memory or event at the same time. Dissociation disconnects memory from memory, memory from consciousness, memory from feeling associated with memory, representations of events from words associated with the event.

Dissociation "can be most simply understood as a self-hypnotic process that attempts to anesthetize and isolate pain. The mind is fleeing its own subjectivity to evacuate pain" (2).

A common example for medical practitioners might be a patient who has had a motor vehicle accident. "What exactly happened?" we ask. Somehow, without loss of consciousness, our patient cannot recall much between his seeing the oncoming car and finding himself sitting by the side of the road, lights flashing in the near distance. It's not that no memory of this event was created, because his consciousness was unbroken. But the totality of the event is too much to be RECREATED right now, for this person. Recalling the danger, the fear, the noise, is more than this person can stand. He may fall silent, stare away. The memory of those moments—the actuality, to the person—is dissociated from current awareness.

"During clinical interviews, dissociation is suggested either by . . . such a degree of unwitting absorption in mental states that ordinary attention . . . is seriously hampered, or by a sudden lack of continuity in discourse, thought or behavior . . . . Thus, for instance, a dissociative patient may suddenly interrupt his or her speech . . . stare into a void for minutes, and become unresponsive to the therapist's queries . . . (or) may suddenly utter fragmented and incoherent comments on intrusive mental images (usually related to the traumatic memories)" (3).

Robert Scaer, a neurologist who worked for much of his career in a rehabilitation setting, writes (4):

> One of the dilemmas of classification of symptoms of dissociation is that these symptoms assume many and varied forms and expressions. They may be emotional, perceptual, cognitive or functional. They may involve altered perception of time, space, sense of self and reality. Emotional expressions may vary from panic to numbing and catatonia. Altered sensory perceptions may vary from anesthesia to analgesia to intolerable pain. Motor expressions frequently involve weakness, paralysis and ataxia, but may also present as tremors, dysarthria, shaking and convulsions. Cognitive symptoms may involve confusion, dysphasia, dyscalculia, and severe deficits in attention. Perceptual symptoms include ignoral (sic) and neglect. Memory alteration may appear as hypermnesia in the form of flashbacks, or as amnesia in the form of fugue states or more selective traumatic amnesia. The varied symptoms of dissociation therefore mimic the intrinsic bipolar nature of the defining symptoms of PTSD (arousal, reexperiencing, avoidance).

Perhaps a person has just lived through a protracted illness and death of a loved one. They come to talk to us about it. They can relay the sequence of medical events without any problem. In fact, they may have many questions about the pathophysiology of their loved one's disease, wondering why this and not that happened? You are the perfect person to answer those questions. What cannot be relayed, what is not now FELT, is the sadness, anger, disgust, resentment, or love the patient may be feeling for their lost relative. It appears not even to be entering the discourse. Those feelings are dissociated. One's patient is not aware of them, does not feel them when reminded they might be present, and would prefer not to get into a discussion about their possible existence. For this person, now, it is safer—less anxiety provoking—to simply put the feelings in a box, shut the lid, and store that box somewhere. Such a person may months later experience a state of inexplicable numbing or depression, be unable to relate it to recent loss, a situation we may label "delayed grief reaction." The dissociated feelings are present but still unlinked to the events that gave them rise.

Dissociation, then, is a last-ditch effort to avoid an overload of unbearable psychic or physical pain. As such, it takes its place in line with such processes as paranoia, denial, and humor as a human way of dealing with the chaos and threatening nature of life. Classically, human defenses are understood as coping mechanisms which keep anxiety at bay. The anxiety may be about something physical—a bear in the kitchen, a father on a rampage; or it may be related to an unwanted emotion or thought. When a beloved parent is also a predator, his child will most likely dissociate in order to avoid the feeling of terror associated with an abandonment or invasion. Dissociation helps us "function," to do what we have to do to survive, with body and some part of mind still "together." It shields the person from the fears associated with annihilation—annihilation of life, of love, of security, of sense of self. It also reduces pain associated with severe physical and mental trauma. It helps animals defend themselves when wounded, it aids soldiers injured on a battleground, and it helps other people living through frightening events to maintain some sense of self-continuity without being "frightened to death."

Dissociation and Medical Practice

Dissociation happens in all kinds of medical settings. We could think here about Elora (Chapter 3), who "wouldn't let me say anything, just KEPT SCREAMING" (at the receptionist). We might understand her behavior around her growing vascular insufficiency as understandable anxiety about an accurate perception of impending disaster. We might understand it as frustration that medical practitioners had not yet understood her problem, perhaps not even believed it; and that in addition, her primary provider (as nascent as our relationship was) was away. Or we might understand someone who KEPT SCREAMING as a rageful, terrified, but defiant child backed into a corner with an abusive father and an overwhelmed, absent mother. What else can such a child do?

I think it is wisest to understand Elora's communications as "all of the above," and more. We need, as medical practitioners, to understand that previous violence is part of this patient's disease. A person who is treating us "violently" may have been treated that way herself, and she is trying to tell us that, even when what happened to her is not yet accessible to memory. She is also yelling at us because she wants us to stop her. She is out of control, as was her abuser. Elora wanted to be able to stop her father, too, but was powerless to do so.

A person who is dissociating is not necessarily violent, although he may have been violated. The key feature is disconnection. For one patient, only a partial memory appears. For another, a catastrophic event is described without emotion; the feelings are dissociated from the information given. For yet another, a physician's reference to something renders a patient speechless. And then, there are the times when a behavior ("SCREAMING") occurs without the person's conscious choice. A frightening experience may be rendered dreamlike. Maybe this didn't really happen to me, is not part of who I am. For the person who is dissociating, things may seem "calm." It is in relationship that the discontinuity surfaces. The clinician must notice, make inquiry, shake off the spell, or, if unsuccessful, get sleepy or experience **in herself** the frightening re-uniting of that which has been isolated and set aside from the stream of her patient's life.

Gabe

I first met Gabe when he was a young man and came for general medical care. He had been married for a few years, was working as an accountant, and was attending classes at night to advance himself. He had graduated from a small, elite college. He complained of toenail fungus, of occasional episodes of proctalgia fugax, dating back 13 years, and of some innocent spots on his scrotum. He was looking forward to having a family at some point in the future. He was soft-spoken and intelligent, often ironically humorous. He told me that he made beer for a hobby (though he only drank one weekly). (Some of Gabe's story has been mentioned briefly in Chapter 2).

On family history, his mother was alcoholic, though, he said, "always under control." His brother? "Very troubled." His father, Gabe told me, was currently beginning to have memories of child sexual abuse at the hands of his own father, Gabe's grandfather. Talking to his dad about these memories was a painful experience, as Gabe had always adored his paternal grandfather. His parents were divorced.

Two years later, he came to be evaluated for what he thought was an allergic reaction to walnuts but sounded like a panic attack, driving home from breakfast out with his wife, now five months pregnant.

A year and half later, he presented with middle insomnia—restlessness, really, which had begun in adolescence. A bit more emerged. Gabe's mother was actually a serious, if closeted, alcoholic. His father had "eventually found out" he was gay, leading to the divorce while Gabe was away at college. He worried a lot about his only (younger) brother, currently "having a series of homosexual affairs." I recall asking Gabe "how did *you* turn out so well?"—which was probably a mistake. I recall his smiling and seeming to understand the question, without really answering it.

His son had been born 15 months earlier and was "a real joy."

We tried him on some amitriptyline for sleep, but it made him gain weight, and he stopped it.

For the next four years, we saw each other only for a variety of minor illnesses.

He then came in with initial insomnia, feeling "trapped," lying awake at night listening to his heart, worrying about work. He now ran his own business, doing accounting for nonprofits. He still had occasional proctalgia. He considered his libido "slightly overreactive" (my notes). His wife wanted him to go on an antidepressant. My notes do not indicate why, or whether Gabe himself met the criteria for depression. We did decide to try citalopram—but he called a month later, worrying about his libido, about interactions with alcohol (he drank one wine nightly). Soon thereafter he stopped it.

Six months later he came with severe lumbar spasm, which has troubled him on and off since. He had also just won a prize for a piece of work he had done, explicating some difficult business concepts. We both felt inordinately pleased, despite his misery with his back. He gave me a signed copy of his piece, though I could not see what it had to do with our work together.

His back improved. He then visited me twice, and a urologist once, about an odd sensation in his groin. No pathology could be found. He gradually became more fit, hiking and doing a regular series of back exercises.

Whenever Gabe would call, it was always with a sense of great need. Messages were marked "URGENT" or "CALL BACK ASAP."

"Gabe," I would say, keeping my mild annoyance (at putting him above someone undressed in the exam room) at bay, "What's up?" "I'm so sorry to trouble you like this, but I need to ask a question," he would answer. There would be a description of a minor event, which we would discuss reasonably, and that was that. Then, "Thank you SO much for your time," he'd say. I could imagine him bowing his head slightly, in acknowledgment, his boyish face alive with gratitude. I adored him.

The real crisis began one summer. Gabe called me while vacationing on a remote island. "I'm wondering if I need to take the next boat home?" he asked. "(His wife) and I have been making love a bit more frequently than usual, and then I felt a 'ping' and now

I see something swollen on the top of my penis!" "What does it look like?" I asked. "It's kind of a pink bump," he said. "Does it hurt?" "No, or maybe slightly. It might itch a little." "How big is it?" "Maybe between a nickel and a dime in diameter." We decided it sounded like a bug bite, a local infection, or perhaps a broken blood vessel. "Gabe, this is a pretty minor thing," I said. "It does not sound like enough to interrupt or end your vacation." He and his family remained on the island as planned. Two weeks later, on his return, all had returned to normal. He wanted to see a second urologist, who found nothing amiss.

Five months later, he presented one week after a startling event. He and his wife had been making love when, during his erection, he began to bleed profusely from his penis. "Cups and cups" of blood, he said. His wife got him an ice pack, and he lay on the floor, bleeding, while she called 911 in the middle of the night. You may be able to imagine Gabe, describing the scene that greeted the firefighters on their arrival. If it had not been frightening, it was at least dramatic. He remained the master of the story! He was transported to the ER in their ambulance "urgently." But, by the time he arrived, the bleeding had settled down to nearly nothing, and he was discharged home. This time, however, he did not lay the subject to rest.

He came in a few days later. Gabe related that he was (and had been for many years) highly inclined toward sexual activity, often masturbating to climax several times daily. He believed that since his brief trial of citalopram, it had been more difficult to reach orgasm, even after stopping the drug (three years before). Out of fear, since the ER visit, he'd been abstinent. It was extremely difficult.

While Gabe spoke to me, I thought about the firefighter's life, ranging from hoses and fires to copious penile hemorrhage. All in a day's work! What had those uniformed men thought and felt as they encountered him? "Gabe," I said, "I have never heard of anything like this!" I was steering us back to his storytelling prowess, something we both enjoyed. I, meanwhile, knew I was out on some sort of limb. Wasn't this "male-only" territory? "I don't think any urologist you see is going to be so familiar with it either," I ventured. "I guess this could be something 'traumatic'—maybe an irritated prostatic urethra? Could this be 'too much' masturbating?" I felt like a Victorian nurse. Why was I even saying this? I had no idea. "You probably should go back to your urologist and have a cystoscopy," I suggested, worrying that maybe there was an anomaly in there, a growth, an AV malformation . . . who knew?

"I'm not sure about that," said Gabe. "It sounds invasive, and painful. I don't think I can do it if I'm awake." I knew he would be, but I said nothing. "Can I go to see (a new urologist, now #3) at (another hospital?) I've heard really wonderful things about him." Who was he talking to about urologists, and why? "I don't think your insurance wants you to go out of network," I said dutifully. Gabe capitulated. What difference would there really be, anyway? None, said my inner cynic. He was just avoiding the inevitable.

A few weeks later, before he went to the local urologist, he had a second, less severe bleed, after resuming relations with his wife. They managed this one at home. It did convince him to attend to himself, and the following week he dragged his feet in to the local urologist. He had the in-office, under-local cystoscopy despite his dread, and some friable tissue was found at his bladder neck and cauterized. Gabe got an antibiotic and instructions about sexual activity.

Gabe came back to see me one month after this visit. He had, after his procedure, emailed the urologist, asking numerous detailed anatomic and pathophysiologic questions. He had cc'd me. They were initially answered by this doctor in a phone call. Later, similar emails, however, went unanswered. The urologist, an experienced and busy man, confided in me that he "couldn't deal with him." Gabe told me he planned to forge ahead with seeing the third urologist. He asked for and got my blessing. Then, we talked some more about his sexuality.

"I had my first orgasm at 11," he told me. Ever since that experience (what **was** that experience, anyway?) "I've had an ongoing, high level of sexual desire. My father and brother were the same way." I wondered to myself how he knew this. Had he learned it contemporaneously, or subsequently?

"Gabe, tell me a little more about what your family was like with you," I inquired. "Oh, they were not that bad," he replied avuncularly, as if trying to soothe me. "My mother was actually pretty far gone in her alcohol addiction by the time I was 15 or so. She insisted on a big, long kiss from me every night, before I went to bed and she passed out. I think it made her feel better. I hated doing it." He ended with his voice gruff and trailing off.

"Your dad?" "My father was gay, but still in the closet and at home before I left for college. He used to masturbate in front of me on various occasions while I was an adolescent." I asked Gabe why he thought his father did this. "I really have no idea," he said thoughtfully, and with a hint of incredulity. He reiterated his worries about his younger brother, who was still quite disturbed and for whose psychiatric care he assured me his dad was paying.

"Gabe," I said, "this may all have seemed like life as normal when you were growing up, but these days, it would be called sexual abuse." "I know that" he said in a clipped voice, as if backed into a corner, but with a humorous edge at the same time. "What do you think is normal male sexual behavior?" Now I was in the corner. What was I supposed to say? I don't really remember what passed for an answer, perhaps that there was an enormous spectrum. I knew I had to get out of answering it and that I didn't really know what he was asking.

"What do you think accompanies your sexual desire, with the wish or drive for orgasms?" I asked. Gabe tried to help me understand. "It's hard to describe, a combination of a physical wish and something mental . . ." His voice again trailed off. He couldn't say more.

We were near the end, for that day. "I'm not sure you are going to be able to continue to live like this," I said. I think maybe your prostate and your urethra are not going to let you. What about exploring more of this with a therapist?" He did not say no.

This was an exhausting conversation, at least for me. It felt like staring at a combination of truth and vulnerability for as long as our relationship could stand. I was able in subsequent days to find him an available therapist with expertise in male abuse, and I gave Gabe his phone number. He was "SO grateful." He did not go.

Gabe did go on to have his specialty evaluation. He emailed me about it: "He found (my condition) startling and recommended a more proactive, thorough approach than Dr. X (urologist #2). I was struck in particular that while he entered our meeting with a similar attitude (dare I call it blasé?), when he heard the extent of the bleeding, he expressed a great deal more concern than Dr. X . . . ." He went on to have blood work, an MRI, and another cystoscopy, this time under general anesthesia, with similar findings. He was again treated with antibiotics.

Six weeks later, Gabe was again asking questions of urologist #3 and getting no reply. He emailed me. "At this point you probably know more about my situation than I do; so far I have only spoken with (the most recent urologist) for perhaps 3 minutes while I was in the recovery room." He cautiously resumed twice a week, "careful" intercourse. He was not satisfied. He has never pursued any psychological treatment.

How Does Recognizing Dissociation Matter?

Outside of practicing medicine in a combat zone, we may not think of violence as a source of human disease. There are so many other things to attend to—diseases of metabolism, of the cardiovascular system, of microbial illness, of neoplasia, and so on. Most of our training has been in understanding the workings of the body as a group of interdependent systems, and the behavior of diseases as they interact with those systems. However, each person is living in a nexus of past and present social situations. More of those situations are violent than we may care to realize (Chapter 2). A good bit of violence is person-on-person, intra-familial, within neighborhoods and in the world.

In 2002, John Stobo and Marla Salmon wrote, for the Institute of Medicine, "[W]e quickly became aware that education of health professionals in family violence is not a consistent priority across or within health professions education curricula. The challenge of even identifying curricular content or strategies was compounded by the almost complete absence of either educational research or evaluation relating to family violence education and training for health professionals. In short, while family violence exacts a tremendous cost from its victims and society, it is not viewed as sufficiently important for society to invest the resources and expertise . . . necessary to improve the response of health professionals and others to this serious social and health problem. That must change" (5).

Recognizing dissociation enables the practitioner to surmise, accept, and work with the trauma history that will often be part of a patient's problem.

A second reason why a working knowledge of dissociation is important is that its presence, both in oneself and in one's patient, hampers one's ability to function fully as a professional. The presence of dissociation may evoke unhelpful, unprofessional responses in providers. These are not our intended responses. They are the human, spoken and unspoken, responses to the situation at hand. They are what we do when we are ignorant, when we are not able to master our emotional responses to a situation, when we are in a hurry, when we have another agenda. They are, in short, responses we have every day. But they are the opposite of professional responses. They are exactly what our dissociating patients do NOT need. As providers, we need to learn how to negotiate this foggy terrain with patients. It is our job to try to understand when dissociation is present, where it is coming from (patient, provider, or system), and to name, with care, the disconnection.

In other words, one of our tasks is to monitor our own mental functioning, to ask ourselves questions about deviations, and to acquire self-awareness. The presence of dissociation in oneself may imply a trauma story somewhere—in the patient, in oneself, in the past, in the present. In engaging with an adult who has had childhood trauma, we become the repository of fragments of a patient's self, and experiences, and our job is to recognize them as such; to allow them to have their effect, to monitor what effect they are having, and then to use them.

Take for example the interactions between Gabe and me as Gabe's narrative unfolded. From his first visit (see Chapter 2) I had fallen under some kind of spell with him. Here I had a delightful, funny, educated man creating for me humorous vignettes of his family life. It was as good as reading a great *New Yorker* article—and right in the middle of a workday! When he came to open up a little more (paragraph 5 of Gabe, above) about his various truths, I went right along with (the adult part of) him. His father had been in the closet for years, then left; his mother was alcoholic; his brother was severely troubled . . . and instead of saying "this could have been troubling for a teenaged boy," I asked him "How did you turn out so well?" We found out years later about the parts of Gabe that were not doing so well—and I foreclosed the opportunity for that to emerge at that time.

I am not saying that Gabe would have told me anything, had my response been different. I know that developing a relationship with a patient who has experienced trauma takes trust and time. What I am saying is that had I known a little more—about dissociation, about myself—I could have reacted, perhaps, more helpfully.

Other examples: Gabe's reaction to cystoscopies, and his urologists' reactions to him. Following two invasive genital procedures, he has multiple questions, becomes persistent, perhaps "urgent," maybe experienced as "overly concerned." To Gabe, his emails and questions seem to flow from the post-op state and an inquiring mind. To me, they sounded like a repetition of some sort; a child seeking solace from the same adult who had inflicted a wound—with no hope of getting it. However, both urologists shut him off and out. An orthopedic surgeon said to me recently, after stating that a hip replacement took only 70 minutes and I expressed surprise, "For a surgeon, the operation starts when he makes the incision and ends with closing." The urologists consider they've done their job, and "can't deal" with *him*—his persistent, driven search for contact with the content subtly disguised. When and how can he go back to his prior sexual behavior? Who or what will answer his needs? Underneath that, what inside of Gabe is driving all of this? His surgeons have no interest in going there. Is it their job to go there? I don't believe they think so. It then falls to the primary physician.

Finally, we as health professionals need to recognize the presence of dissociation and know about the traumas in our patient's lives, because it makes a difference. This is not to say that we are therapists. We refer our troubled patients to therapists and wish them well on that hard journey. Many do not, or cannot, go. Of those who do, we usually don't hear a lot about it. The point is that we are **not** referring the problem away, nor do we lack a role. If we know what has gone on, or if we have an inkling, shared or not, that trauma has occurred, we are in a position to help—more than we know. Many people who dissociate are incredibly tuned in to us. Often, if we suspect something, they know that we do. It may not be spoken for years, or ever. One picks one's times. But it affects how we act with them, and certainly how we advocate for them. It affects how they feel about us and grow to trust us. Such awareness on both of our parts confers a measure of wholeness on our patients, who can be both themselves AND their dissociated part-selves and experiences, with us. All parts of the self have an audience. All are tended to. All are believed. At times, one is in the rare and privileged position to be one of a few—sometimes the only—person who gets to help someone in this way.

The Brain and Dissociation

In the past 40 years or so, psychological healers have again begun to acknowledge the existence of trauma in the lives of their patients. With this "new" knowledge, both the concept of dissociation and awareness of its manifestations have become more present for clinicians. As luck would have it, this reawakening has occurred along with the development of techniques for imaging and understanding the brain as one (but perhaps not only) physical reservoir of mind. We now have the voices and tools of experts from the fields of psychology, neurology, neurobiology, and human development weighing in on dissociation.

Scaer (6) defines mind as "a perceptual experience, generated by a complex set of synapses, neurons, and neurochemical states and determined by genes, instinct and experience, that is capable of developing and directing novel behavior." Noting that brain, mind, and body are a continuum, each capable of messaging and influencing the others, he explores trauma as an experience generating the survival behaviors of fight or flight. When the (human) animal realizes that these are not working, they often then "freeze"—playing "possum." "This freeze response, common to all species, indeed may allow the animal to survive, but in mammals it sometimes comes at a terrible cost. Animals who survive the freeze response experience an unconscious 'discharge' of all the energy and stored memories of the threat and failed escape through stereotyped body movements as the animal 'awakens'. If they don't experience this discharge, a host of adverse behavioral and health problems may follow."

Scaer distinguishes declarative or explicit memory, which he localizes to the hippocampus and is associated with conscious learning, from procedural, implicit memory, stored in the "reptilian" brain—sub-tentorial territory, which is separated from consciousness and brings about learned behaviors that are involved in survival. Explicit memory is subject to decay; implicit memory is remarkably resistant to it. Implicit memory serves us well in learning important skills in day-to-day situations (removing hand from fire, riding a bicycle) and encodes, as well, the emotions and sensory experiences that accompany this learning. All of this happens through conditioning. When learning happens during a threatening situation, however, implicit memory "becomes a source of confusion of the past and the present. . . In unresolved traumatic stress, procedural memory turns inward, responding to internal cues of a threat that no longer exists, evoking inappropriate somatic and autonomic experiences and responses that pertain to cues unwittingly emerging from past memory rather than from present external experiences."

When, due to inferior size or wounding, an animal (or child) cannot effectively fight or flee, it freezes—becomes immobile, collapses, "feigns death." Scaer comments on the autonomic instability of the freeze response—both sympathetic and parasympathetic nervous systems are active and alternating. "The animal in freeze is in a precarious state of abnormally dysregulated and fluctuating autonomic nervous system activity. . . . The perceptual experience at that moment is called dissociation. It is physiologically the same as the freeze." He comments on the tendency of the freeze to be accompanied by an endorphin response, which may condition the organism to return to freezing, during future threats.

He goes on to discuss Porges' theory of the dorsal vagal complex, present in reptiles and mammals and governing the parasympathetic response during a freeze, and which, if overly active or prolonged in mammals may be implicated in sudden cardiovascular death. Mammals also have a ventral vagal complex, which modulates this discharge but can be overridden by severe threat and prolonged freeze. He then presents Levine's work based on his theory of the importance of the "freeze discharge"—and involving completing "the motor discharge of the freeze through unique behavioral therapeutic techniques. In the absence of this freeze discharge, the 'energy' of the intense arousal associated with the threat and attempted escape, remains bound in body and brain, leading to a host of abnormal symptoms that we attribute to PTSD. . . . The key to this dilemma of inhibited discharge seems to lie in the attainment of empowerment, freedom, and ultimately completion."

I recommend Dr. Scaer's book for a more through explication of the brain and body in trauma, one that is relevant to general, non-neurologic practice. His understanding of the neurobiology of dissociation shows both its positive and negative effects, again highlighting the importance of recognizing and working with our patients who use it. While we will not be involved in behavioral or other psychotherapies, it is certainly important to work with our patients on releasing them from disempowerment.

Wilkinson (7), striving to integrate Jungian concepts with neuroscience, says:

> Early brain development is adversely affected by traumatic experiences in the earliest relationships. Teicher's research has shown the impaired connections between the right and left hemispheres, that the fibre tract known as the corpus callosum, that is the major highway between the two hemispheres, may be reduced through the effects of trauma in those who have experienced childhood sexual abuse . . . Schore has brought together evidence from a substantial body of research, including research using EEG and neuro-imaging (fMRI) data and positron emission topography (PET), that demonstrates that unconscious processing of emotion is associated with the right rather than the left hemisphere and that the right hemisphere is densely interconnected with limbic regions and therefore contains the major circuitry of emotion regulation. In (a) recent paper Schore stresses the importance of the "hierarchical vertical cortico-subcortical functions"

> of the right brain and argues that dissociation is best understood, not in terms of disconnection of left and right brains, but in terms of a loss of connectivity within the right hemisphere. . . . For our dissociative patients it is important that we engage the right brain in an empathic mode of working towards relational change but whilst crucially remaining able to think.

Clearly, the neuroanatomy of dissociation remains an active topic for research. The brain is the elephant, and we are blind women and men groping tail and trunk. These explorations, however, lay a basis for engaging with our patients. We have come to see that dissociation is not just a defense mechanism in the lives of trauma survivors. It has become a part of their neural architecture, as the fear response did in PTSD. If trauma or neglect happened early enough, long enough, or was intense enough, the survivor's brain and nervous system has changed. It is less supple, more rigid, prone to flooding and fixating on the past, and prey to autonomic and attendant immune dysfunction, earlier disease, and death.

In addition, many trauma survivors have gone for 5, 10, 20 or more years living their lives, learning and working as best as they can and involved in their relationships, with altered neurophysiology. They, and others, know themselves to be the way they are. When we encounter such people, either with medical problems or life problems, including the problems that their dissociated parts engender, we will be meeting all parts of them.

As we think about our next patient, Marta, let's return to one definition: "Dissociation as a clinical . . . condition has been defined primarily in terms of the fragmentation and splitting of the mind, and perception of the self and the body. Its clinical manifestations include altered perceptions and behavior, including derealization, depersonalization, distortions of perception of time, space and body, and conversion hysteria" (8).

Marta

I took care of Marta for over 22 years, starting in her early 40s. She and her family had come to this country legally from Central America when she was a young child. She'd grown up as an American, done a stint in the military after high school, then gone to college at night while working. She married briefly after her time in the service, but when I knew her she was divorced and single. Marta was now a middle manager in a large corporate setting. She first came because an oral surgeon had wanted her to be checked before having her wisdom teeth taken out. She alluded, during that brief visit, to having pelvic pain, and eventually returned a year later for a longer exam. She complained of urinary urgency, especially after sexual relations. We talked about whether her diaphragm was the right size, and she was ultimately referred to a gynecologist to have a cervical cap fit.

Over the next three to four years her main complaints, if she had any, were of intermittent dull right-sided abdominal or flank pain, which would come and go, often fleetingly. One night she developed a high fever, came to the hospital, and was found to have a raging right-sided pyelonephritis. Imaging studies did not reveal stone or obstruction, but her pain subsided very slowly; she required a longer than usual hospital stay; and even at discharge she was not pain-free, though her infection was gone.

For the next year, Marta had right-sided abdominal pain of two types, both different from her initial, transitory pains. One was under her ribs, ranging from "noticeable to screaming"; one was deeper and came on with digestion, driving, or before moving her bowels. Palpation of her colon in her right upper quadrant reproduced the second pain. She saw me, and went as well to several different gastroenterologists, whom she picked out. I only heard from one. Contrast x-rays were normal. The local GI consultant told me it was "all functional bowel syndrome." During one of her visits, she let me know that her mother had died "mysteriously" of cancer at the age of 42, when Marta was 10 years old. She was not told at the time what was wrong with her mother, though she had noticed her "dwindling," she said, and her death was a complete shock. Marta was now in the same decade her mother had been when she died.

After a while Marta seemed to stop going to all her consultants, and me. Months later when she did return, her colon pain seemed better on no specific treatment, but the "screaming" rib pain was not. She was angry, tearful, and "desperate." Exam was unchanged. Stalling for time, I tinkered with meds, ordered rib films (normal), and thought about our conversation regarding her mother. I asked her, hesitantly, if she would be amenable to a psychological evaluation, and she was. She agreed to a four-visit consultation. I sent her to someone with whom I had worked previously with other patients who were somewhere on the mind-body continuum. The psychologist called me at the end of the four visits, enumerated current issues in Marta's life, noted she had "trouble communicating anger," and said she had recommended ongoing treatment, which Marta declined.

I had no idea how to connect "trouble communicating anger" and rib pain.

Nine months later, a note from the psychologist indicated that Marta had reconnected over a crisis with a friend. As part of that, she went to a psychopharmacologist, who suggested amitriptyline—which got rid of both of her pains! She saw me seven months later and confirmed this. Now, she was mostly concerned about upcoming menopause, including fears of "uncontrollable and unbearable" premenstrual symptoms.

Several years ensued. Then she brought us a new complaint—vaginal burning, "10 years" of urinary urgency and frequency, about which I had only heard sporadic mention, though I had been seeing her for those same 10 years. WHAT? I thought. Have I been forgetting something? Or ignoring something? Looking over all my notes, I could not find an ongoing 10-year complaint like this. Yet, Marta told me, she had already visited two urologists (whom I did not know) and had a workup of whose results she was unclear. I sent for their records, which contained only a set of negative urinalyses and cultures. I asked her what these urinary symptoms were linked to. She thought "stressful situations" caused some of her symptoms. My examination of her, including a pelvic exam, was negative. Her bowel complaints now waxed and waned at a low level.

A year later she saw one of the urologists, who did a flexible cystoscopy in the office due to intermittent flank pain, and microscopic hematuria. He called me (an unusual event), noting that the patient had been in severe pain during the procedure. The exam was unremarkable. I called Marta to commiserate, but I didn't see her or hear from her after that for a couple of years.

Late in this interval I was out on maternity leave for four months. While I was away, she asked that her urology records be sent to yet a third urologist, and she also sent me a 10-page hand-printed letter. Writing, I have since learned, is not unusual for trauma patients. It is often easier to relate by phone or written word. Neither of us were there, but the communication was hanging "in the air," so to speak, and the dissociation is in our physical absence from each other.

In the letter she detailed now "30 years" of bladder and urethral pain, and her many interactions with urologists and gynecologists. Topical Premarin, which I had prescribed three years earlier but did not know if she had used, now caused "hideous, unbearable pain . . . like a raging, weeping sore." Upon my return, Marta came in, and we had numerous long, detailed and complex in-person and phone consults. She'd been worse for eight months. She had been given antibiotics for "urinary tract infections," one of which caused an ER visit where drug-induced hepatitis was diagnosed, felt to be related to Bactrim. She again noted problems with topical Premarin. She had been to several gynecologic and urology providers, none of whom had sent me any notes. I felt overwhelmed by all Marta's unconfirmed interactions with specialists. The lack of records made it impossible for me to develop a cohesive picture and plan.

Ultimately one of the urologists diagnosed her with interstitial cystitis, after another cystoscopy. I asked Marta to obtain these records, and she did, and sent them to me. She also questioned the diagnosis, as by now, she said, she had mainly (severe) urethral pain. Other, previously mentioned symptoms had disappeared somewhere. She and I considered an estrogen patch. She saw a neurologist, who noted she had a normal exam and suggested more amitriptyline. I wrote to Wyeth about their experience with topical Premarin reactions ("rare spontaneous reports"). Her new urologist suggested dimethyl sulfoxide (DMSO) infusions into her bladder, after first seeing a pain specialist to get her "pain under control." I laughed to myself at that wish. Marta saw yet another (tertiary) urologist, who specialized in interstitial cystitis, and he recommended against DMSO. I spoke with the diagnosing urologist. How could he explain her predominantly urethral symptoms? He told me that he thought her urethral pain was due to her bladder inflammation, and said he was thinking also about steroids, or perhaps a cystectomy if the DMSO did not work. How frightening and extreme a thought was that??

Marta opted to try the DMSO. The trial occurred over a number of months. It was not very successful, giving her mild relief of mild bladder urgency but continued urethral pain. She again wrote me about the pain late in the treatment . . . "like someone is POUNDING up there as HARD AS CAN BE!!! (like a rape)." It was time for me to see her again. Marta came. Had she ever been assaulted? At 16 she had had a bad snowboard accident, in which the board came up and hit her right between the legs. She had been seen then by a local doctor who told her she would eventually be fine. She denied any other trauma, including molestation or rape. We again debated trying an estrogen patch.

She was losing a lot of work time due to her symptoms.

As the DMSO trial came to a close, Marta went to a GI consultant, whom she saw twice for queasiness and morning feverishness and dizziness. Where had those symptoms come from? This consultant noted and listed the 18 drugs she'd been given over the course of the last few months, none of which had helped any of her symptoms. Reading the list gave me a tiny bit of welcome relief. Someone else had noticed the discoordination between physicians, each acting insularly—dissociated from each other. In addition, this doctor told me, Marta complained of feeling toxic, as if there was something in her system which was poisoning her. The gastroenterologist suggested a "therapist of sorts to help deal with the chronic illness." She also suggested two endoscopic studies, neither of which the patient pursued. I, meanwhile, trying to catch up, spoke with the pain consultant recommended months ago by the DMSO urologist. "She needs a psychopharmacologist," he said to me. People, I thought, I've been trying to go there with Marta for years.

I somehow knew that I had to be Marta's "glue." I tried, always feeling tardy and disorganized, to catch up with all the providers she visited, all the hints she gave me. It was a messy, incomplete job. Maybe she returned to me to provide whatever cohesiveness she was ready for and that I could provide—a poor substitute for psychic wholeness. If I ever put aside how she was suffering, she came back to remind me about that, too.

Early the following year, Marta and I decided to try the estrogen patch after her (interstitial cystitis) urologist tried a hypogastric nerve block, which did not alleviate her symptoms. The estrogen helped a great deal at first, but there were problems with bleeding, dosing, and incomplete response, and I referred her to another gynecologist, with whom she formed a good relationship. After some months, she experienced disappointment with her only partially remitted symptoms. A hoped-for intimate relationship with a man ended when she was unable to tolerate intercourse. An intermittent dental problem and antibiotics caused esophagitis and a vaginal yeast infection, with flare of her pain. By the end of the year, she was "very discouraged . . . extremely distraught." She'd had to take a demotion and a pay cut at work, due to her health issues.

Because of the complexity of her case, I wrote a summary of the 18 months of treatment, not wanting to leave pieces out. I had the following experience:

> As I write this, I become overwhelmed with the need to close my eyes and float away—sleep somewhere. This is a feeling I get from time to time when talking to patients, when the monotonous complaints and the relentless nature of their voice or their suffering overwhelms me. I am the numbing board for their feelings. And what is it which would wake me up? The truth, perhaps, but it looms much too great for whatever we have between us—which is "here is the person who has to listen to me and is getting paid to do it" and "here comes this person who has persistent complaints and doesn't get better, who is tortured and tortures me, here she comes" . . . that's what's between us. I have to go sit and sleep, and my head swims with indefinable images, I can't reproduce them, I have to get away from them and sink down for a while. . . . There is also the confusion. Trying to sort out all the facets—having so many people recommend trying so many different things, keeping the threads going . . . and at some point, it is too much. Especially since the patient won't tell you what they were supposed to try and didn't, and can't say why they didn't do it, and yet it is my job to keep track, even though the patient can't, and that gets overwhelming too.

Meanwhile, Marta had heard about a new drug, Elmiron, marketed for interstitial cystitis, and wanted to try it. Inwardly, I was skeptical. Another treatment, another disappointment, for something that both of us were unsure that she had. Really? "Before trying this," I said, "let's get yet another opinion." I sent her to another urologist I had worked with 20 years earlier when we were both young, energetic, and idealistic. I also wrote to Baker Norton Pharmaceuticals to get information about Elmiron, which appeared to be harmless and seemed to provide a modest benefit to a small but significant number of people with interstitial cystitis.

After records were sent, she saw the urologist. I got a prompt letter from him, and prompt follow-up, also, from Marta.

(Dr. Y) felt many of her symptoms were atypical for interstitial cystitis; he reviewed her lack of progress with DMSO, and some progress with hormone replacement. "After quite a lengthy conversation, I came to the following conclusions: One I thought it was reasonable to start her on low dose valium as a skeletal muscle relaxant, since most of her symptoms sounded like a tight pelvic floor. Two I'm not absolutely sure that any of her symptoms are coming from her bladder at the moment, though I did suggest that we might be able to prove that with a cystometrogram. She was not too excited about any manipulation at this time, so I let it go." He prescribed low dose valium and asked for a call-back. "She also mentioned that she was interested in Elmiron therapy, which of course, is available, although has not seemed to do very much for this disorder."

(Letter from Marta, penned that same evening): "His opinion was that a straight diagnosis of interstitial cystitis just doesn't fit. He said that labeling my condition 'painful bladder syndrome' was a lot more accurate than calling it IC. . . . The major points that struck him (and have always bothered me, too) are the facts that I don't have real urgency; don't have to go to the bathroom, literally, every 15 minutes. . . . I don't have to get up several times during the night . . . my pain seems to be very low in my pelvic and vulvar area, and not necessarily in the bladder, but often over all my pelvic area . . . and the fact that, although estrogen, theoretically, does absolutely nothing for IC, it helped me significantly. . . . He thought it was significant that my pain pretty much disappears when I am in a tub of hot water . . . this, of course, indicates that relaxing those muscles alleviates the pain."

I had never heard her say that *anything* completely relieved her pain. How nice to finally know this! On the other hand, this letter felt like the healthiest, most "integrated" note from Marta that I had ever received. Her mind was clear, and her personhood was present, too.

"By the way, he is the FIRST urologist I have seen (and I've seen a total of six, including him, since this problem started) that actually LISTENS to what I am describing and then thinks through what THAT might mean instead of just proclaiming a pat this or that answer. I think he may be a little puzzled as to a total answer to explain ALL of my symptoms, and that is good because he not only believes that I have the type of location of pain and discomfort that cannot be fully explained and solved by some IC 'formula,' but he is aware that to help me, he's got to look beyond IC 'formulas.' The fact that he is very personable doesn't hurt either, so thank you very much for referring me to him."

I did not see Marta, or hear anything about her pain, for 18 months. Then, she appeared for an annual exam. She was now having problems with workplace harassment. She had had a hip injury, and in doing physical therapy had re-injured her perineal area. Despite this, her urethral complaints were markedly reduced on a regime of Estraderm patch and Provera. She was continuing to be followed by the same gynecologist with whom she had begun treatment when the first estrogen patch trial went awry. She was also going to a therapist close to her home. She had uncovered further memories of her childhood. Marta looked directly into my eyes, and said quietly, "You were right, there was some abuse back then." Her father had been brutally physically violent with her and her siblings as children. She was taking a low dose of imipramine. Her urethral symptoms had vastly improved. She felt much of her relief was due to estrogen supplementation. Despite Marta's growing conscious awareness of her past, she was most comfortable with a physical explanation of her suffering. And menopause was most definitely a part of it.

Nothing ends simply. One could hope that with this sort of breakthrough, Marta's miseries would begin to abate. However, we continued to work over the years with musculoskeletal pain, headaches, crawling sensations, months of morning queasiness and nausea, and periodic debilitating and lengthy recurrences of urethral pain. Problems also continued for several years with her boss, whom she described as "verbally violent" and harassing, despite mediation done with her HR department. She continued in psychotherapy. From time to time, she filled me in on more of her childhood as well. She had had this same queasiness every morning as a child, wondering what her father would be up to. Her father had beaten her and her siblings from her toddlerhood to age 18, when she left home for good. She had lived intermittently with relatives after her mother's death. She did not know why, or how. She had tried despite her father's behavior to seek praise and recognition from him.

Months later, Marta came in to tell me that in reality, her mother had not had cancer at all. She had shot herself, when Marta was 10, inside the family home. Marta had been out of the house at the time with other family, who told her incidentally, later in the day.

Dissociation Revisited

For 16 years, the psychological component and origins of Marta's illness were absent from our joint view. As in the case of Gabe, however, she had hinted at them in our first visit, while seeking clearance for dental extractions—or perhaps I should say dental distraction. This, in retrospect, was my first clue that dissociation was operative.

Recovery from her pyelonephritis was problematic, with longer than usual pain. This problem evolved into two and a half years of pain syndromes related to the same area but caused by "something else." One pain was prolonged and became "screaming, deep inside." **Altered sensory perceptions may vary from anesthesia to analgesia to intolerable pain.** We got a little closer with the prolonged bout of urethral pain, which was so refractory to diagnosis and prompted so much confusion, theorizing, medications, and exams. The pain was "like someone is POUNDING up there as HARD AS CAN BE!!! (like a rape)." Memory of the snowboard injury surfaced but nothing else, yet. **Memory alteration may appear as hypermnesia in the form of flashbacks, or as amnesia in the form of fugue states or more selective traumatic amnesia.** Was Marta **uttering fragmented and incoherent comments on intrusive mental images?** In trying to understand what was going on, getting the sequence, I found myself dissociating. I could hardly stay awake and recalled times when other patients' recitations had caused me to go numb as well. **Its presence, in oneself or one's patient, affects one's ability to function as a professional.** Memory recall for Marta was slow, piecemeal, and not usually liberating. Life mimicked parts of her past. There were situations she was stuck with that could not be realistically changed, though she tried.

My job, during these many years, was to try to provide a steady hand on the tiller. Marta's suffering was loud, clear, and inexplicably shifting. From the first, I had had my questions. I tried to listen, non-judgmentally, both to her and to the various specialists, including providers with seemingly ludicrous or misguided, ill-timed ideas. I tried as best I could to track down the pieces of her story kept in cocoons, here and there. I felt determined, but often overwhelmed. I got bogged down in my own dissociation, trying to put it all together. Dissociation really is a contagious condition.

It is in understanding and interacting with our trauma-surviving patients that the educated generalist can be at the peak of his powers. Such a clinician can not only diagnose and differentiate between clot and vasospasm, between prostatitis and cancer. He must also stand at the juncture of the anatomic and the functional, the land of understood physiology, the land of front-line neurophysiology, and the land of his own living intuition. He must lead the way in helping patient, self, and specialist integrate it all. He can believe everything from the patient's point of view and help to soothe her; he can finely tune his observational skills so that he knows what he himself must believe; and he can help everyone decide when to go forward with an investigation and when to hold off. He can help the patient profit from helpful procedural encounters and can believe the patient—and help her process—about those that are not helpful. He can periodically reflect with the patient on hints the patient herself gives about her development. He can also stand ready to help his specialist colleagues understand different dimensions of a patient's pain because some parts of him, and some parts of his patient, know more—so much more—about where the suffering really comes from.

References

1. Patient, private communication, 1998.
2. Schwartz HL, "From dissociation to negotiation, a relational psychoanalytic perspective on multiple personality disorder," *Psychoanalytic Psychology* 11(1): 189–231; quoted in Bromberg P, *Standing in the Spaces*, p. 190, The Analytic Press, 1998.
3. Liotti G, "Trauma, dissociation, and disorganized attachment: three strands of a single braid," *Psychotherapy: Theory, Research, Practice, Training* 9(4): 472–486, 2004.
4. Scaer R, "The neurophysiology of dissociation and chronic disease," in David Baldwin's *Trauma Information Pages*, www.trauma-pages.com, Eugene, Oregon. See also Dr. Scaer's excellent book, *The Trauma Spectrum: Hidden Wounds and Human Resiliency*, WW Norton, 2005, pp. ix–x.

5. Cohn F, Salmon ME, and Stobo JD, eds., *Confronting Chronic Neglect: The Education and Training of Health Professionals on Family Violence*, Institute of Medicine, National Academy Press, Washington, DC, 2002, pp. ix–x.
6. Scaer R, *The Trauma Spectrum, Hidden Wounds and Human Resiliency*, WW Norton, 2005.
7. Wilkinson M, "Undoing dissociation. Affective neuroscience: a contemporary Jungian clinical perspective," *Journal of Analytical Psychology* 50(4): 483–501, 2005.
8. Scaer R, "The neurophysiology of dissociation," 2005.

5

Power and Control

In general, we keep our power when we protect the power of others (1). *Good (treatment) conveys a belief in the person's ability to deal with and if necessary, change what is . . . Good treatment and good treaters are not born out of the pages of countless volumes of per se professional books, but (are) born out of the outcomes of numerous interactions with persons who are what these professionals want to know. The treater is (if open) taught by his patient what is and how to's of treating.* (Val, v.i.)

Introduction

A search of the medical literature on the subject of power reveals scant results. Yet the clinician's use (or abuse) of her powers is critical to the outcome of much that is done in medicine. Physicians spend years acquiring the medical knowledge, skills, and judgment needed to act wisely in the face of disease. Good doctors continue to refine and expand their knowledge base throughout their career. An effective clinician must also learn to create a "safe space" for patients as they reveal themselves and confront disease and the unknown. Finally, a good healer tasks herself to learn from vulnerability and disease along with each patient.

The use of power for good or ill is of particular concern to the patient who has survived a traumatic past. Such a patient has been on the receiving end of abusive power and has become, for survival reasons, attuned to its presence. He may not be verbal, or even conscious, about his intuition but will nevertheless have a reaction to it. It is likely that the treating clinician will be made aware of this reaction sooner or later.

Such patients will also have understandable difficulty trusting that "good power" is being offered, even when it is. Their early trust was violated, and often their understanding of the very nature of trust is also confused. In addition, none of us (patients included) is perfect. There may be traces of self-aggrandizement, humiliation, or minimization in anything clinicians do, even with the best of training, intentions, and character.

Perhaps most importantly, violence and neglect by their very nature degrade a victim's sources of personal power. Trauma survivors often have eroded souls. Fear and neglect undermine one's beliefs, principles, hopes, and trust—not just in others but also in oneself and in one's sources of spiritual strength. Survivors therefore enter the medical "playing field" facing a more uneven balance of power than most. This is one reason some choose not to enter the arena at all, or do so only under great duress. If and when they do come, such patients may tend to feel overpowered and unskilled. They may also place undue weight on the clinician's words or wishes at the expense of their own.

A healing relationship must strive to repair this breach. It is no small task.

Abusive Power

All humans are born with power, and powers. Growing up is, in part, an education in using one's powers for the purpose of getting one's needs and desires met. Examples abound: babies cry; toddlers explore; children whine and cajole; older children argue; teenagers deceive. As children mature, their knowledge of their own power, their repertoire, and their opportunities for its use all expand toward the goal of independent and interdependent adulthood.

A young person who has been sexually or physically violated or neglected has had a shocking experience with loss of power and self-authority. Superimposed on the stream of normal development has been one or many episodes of powerlessness. The young person's boundaries of self and body are violated for the gratification or service of another, usually a bigger, stronger, more resourceful other or others. The messages are clear: your life is in danger if you do not do what I want; you may be miserable now, but I can make it worse; there is no one here to help you; your body is mine to play with; I can lie to the world and be believed, you can tell the truth and you will be ridiculed; what you think is happening is just in your mind; you count only as you are available to me. This is a situation, time-limited or not, in which the world colludes with the abuser and not with the child. The abuser's messages about lies, truth-telling, and ridicule are all too often backed up by what happens when children attempt enlist others' help.

People who serve in the military are also vulnerable to abusive power, particularly during wartime. Of necessity, one surrenders one's personal will to the group command. This can lead to personal growth and strength, but the very nature of war—killing of other humans, "collateral damage" to civilians, witnessed suffering, and the unleashing of evil—subjects people to forces for which none of us could be prepared. Wartime trauma may also erode a young person's sense of personal potency, self-efficacy, and moral outlook.

Such experiences involve coercion, shaming, and silencing. The coercion may be via threat and pain, as in a rape or beating, or via grooming and withholding, as in seduction by a father or camp counselor; or it may involve voluntary consent, as in military service. Shame, which as observers we would assign to the perpetrator,* is always experienced by the victim. Shame can come from what was done to the young person, or what he felt he should have done but did not, or could not. Silencing is usually easy.

Children with abusive relatives are told they should never tell—they won't be believed, or more of the same will be visited upon them, or they will bring down their families, and so on. Defense lawyers are skilled at undermining the character of rape victims in court. Society colludes with veterans to keep them silent about their real experiences, in the name of heroism.

Even experiences not involving overt violence—for instance, confrontations with exhibitionists, public fondling, exposure to misogynist behavior and the like, disempower victims by taking place in the context of "normal" activity between humans. Suddenly, a child is face to face with a person deliberately singling her out, using his gestures or words to insult her, while life proceeds normally around her. A student can be mocked in front of classmates by a teacher exposing his deficiencies. These are hateful acts.

Eyewitness accounts bring the above to life.

A father assaults his two young daughters:

> Our beds were next to each other. He would sit me on my bed and say, "Now watch very carefully. Watch what happens to little girls who think nasty thoughts." Then he would . . . he would do these (whispered) horrible things to her . . . I didn't even know what he was doing then. Now, I know. She would cry out for help. It must have hurt her terribly (crying now). No one ever came. I never understood where my mother was, why she never came. It didn't feel real. I used to think to myself, if this is real, why doesn't Mommy come. He told me that if I ever told anyone what I saw, he would do the same things to me; then he would tell them that I was crazy, and they would come and lock me up in a mental hospital. He said I must never speak about it at all. Of course, I obeyed. For a while.

(The child learned to feign sleep, or actually would fall asleep during these paternal visits).

* Perpetrators themselves have often been victims

> There seemed to be no retaliation for this. It was probably a relief to have me out of the way. The odd thing though, was waking up in the morning. It was as if I was waking from a bad dream. Everything was just as it had been the night before when I went to bed. Everyone was normal; my father, my mother . . . just the way they always were; but nothing like the way they were at night. I would think, he couldn't possibly have done such things; she couldn't have allowed such things to go on. . . . Then I would be sure that I had made the whole thing up. I would think how hideously evil I must be to invent such thoughts about my own loving parents (2).

The lessons of abusive power are lessons about the self and others. People are not who they seem. Those who are bigger, stronger, entrusted with me, can arbitrarily change identity and hurt me for inexplicable reasons. They can believe and convince others that they are doing this because *I* am bad. (The abuser's evil is projected on to the victim/observer). If I complain, I, or someone I love, will be annihilated/eliminated. If I act on my anger, I endanger myself and others. *I had best not know the anger is there.* If I believe my eyes and memory, I fly in the face of what I love and need. Because I saw and lived through this, and did nothing, I am just as bad as the perpetrator.

A GI witnesses a gang rape:

> While I was on the base taking care of KIAs (Killed in Action) as they came through, I made friends with people in my company that I considered basically nice people. We used to get together at night and talk. I went down to a certain place where they all were and as I approached it, I heard a scream. Someone was obviously very scared. As I got down to the door, I called one of my friends. He punched this chick on the side of the head. The girl was, you know, Vietnamese people are a lot smaller than American people. It doesn't take that much to hurt one of those people, you know? They gave her a couple of good shots and the girl finally started yelling, "me do, me do, me do," and about seven of them ripped her off. I know the guys, and I know basically they're not really bad people, you know? I just couldn't figure out what was going on to make the people like this do it. It was just part of the everyday routine.
>
> —Specialist/4 Timon Hagelin, testifying to Congress about his service in the American war effort in Vietnam, 1968–1969 (3)

Later testimony by many GIs confirmed the "everyday routine" of sexual exploitation and murder of Vietnamese children, teenagers, and adults by bands of roving GIs, including during the infamous massacre at My Lai.

What did that South Vietnamese adolescent, a victim of gang rape at the hands of the supposedly aiding US military, learn about power? She learned that she could easily choose to give her body away when threatened with torture or death. She learned the terror of a captive. She learned about the duplicity of humans. She learned how little she, herself, mattered. Even to a sympathetic listener, her fate was "everyday routine." She could easily have learned the "everyday" emotional lessons of abuse: shame, self-loathing, isolation, helplessness, and rage.

The GI witness incorporated some of the same knowledge. In the face of atrocity (dead buddies are "KIAs") discipline breaks down; stated goals and behaviors disappear; those in power look the other way; if I act, I may be shamed or overpowered; if I do not act I become part of this victimization forever; somehow I must normalize this as "everyday routine." The GI's humanity suffers; and cynicism about lofty goals, and the personnel entrusted with them, takes firm root and grows.

Medical Power and Its Limits

Providers spend years acquiring the knowledge and skill needed to be responsible for and to patients. As they take increasing responsibility for people's health, they need also to learn the art and science of effective relationship-building. These are valid sources of power. Other sources exist. These pertain to medicine's social roles and connections and are something practitioners may take for granted. But they may be felt implicitly by patients of all sorts. Power inheres in the institution of medicine in society. Medical professionals are seen as experts on how the health of individuals and populations is to be secured, and they have empowered leaders and representatives to maintain and buttress that power locally and nationally. Doctors and physician extenders make more money than the average individual. In America, and likely elsewhere, this matters. Many doctors have grown up in positions of privilege, in families who can afford the expensive educations they must acquire. Many doctors expect to provide the same for their own children. Without trying, they exude a sense of power, and often they enjoy it.

All people entering the medical system—providers and patients—are forced to adjust to the power dynamics of the medical encounter. Each encounter is, among many other things, a request by the patient (for services), and an acknowledgment by the patient of vulnerability (to disease, aging, ignorance, bad habits, uncertainty). So, the very **act** of doctoring sets up a power disparity between doctor and patient. The doctor's training and knowledge, along with social reinforcements, add to the inequality. It is best for a clinician to be aware and sometimes explicit that there is a power differential basic to the relationship and the enterprise.

When done well, doctoring also harnesses the powers of love, attention, altruism, professionalism, personal growth, connectedness, and skill. In a flourishing primary care relationship, patient and doctor can use some or all these attributes in the service of the patient. Both benefit: the patient heals and adjusts; the doctor grows in skill and compassion.

Most doctors have some insight into the need for trust-building at the commencement of and during a medical relationship. For a survivor of child abuse, trust is not just a nicety. Trust and a sense of safety are essential for the accomplishment of *anything*. Trust and safety must be established; this is the clinician's first task. Building a safe place with the patient often means allowing the survivor to have a good deal of leeway in establishing the terms of the relationship. Encountering this essential need alters the usual paradigm of the doctor–patient relationship and can cause a lot of confusion and misunderstanding. It can seem just plain "weird." It causes both physician and patient to wonder just what is going on.

The goal of training is the wise use of our powers; it is one basis of the good we can do and of professional satisfaction and growth. Listening well, doing a thorough and sensitive exam, choosing tests and consultants wisely, thinking broadly and deeply, doing a complex procedure well, using intuition—all of these are skills and powers a good clinician refines throughout his career. Patient empowerment is embedded in many of these proficiencies. Most clinicians educate, correct misperceptions, explore options, and negotiate decisions with patients daily.

Because of their previous, often shattering encounters with abusive power, abuse and neglect survivors have, intelligently, become extremely wary about the exercise of power and the experience of powerlessness, as it pertains to them. Empowerment of themselves, the honest and explicit use of power for their benefit, and a delineation of limits are the opposite of what they have learned about power, somewhere in the marrow of their being. The presence of power reminds them of the depth and pain of loss of agency. Experiencing a powerful presence may evoke only their loss of faith in this world where right and wrong have been confusingly enmeshed or upended. Personal vulnerability has led to exploitation. People who enjoy their own power are best avoided.

Several initial tasks must be undertaken before such a patient and doctor can begin to make use of medical power. For some, these tasks may take one or several sessions; for others, their accomplishment takes years. For most dyads, the work must be returned to again and again. These initial and ongoing endeavors include the building of trust and the nurture of the patient's personal powers, which have become warped, hidden, or completely lost.

Trust

The building of trust involves honesty, respect, integrity, and repair of inevitable breaches. Trust does not require perfection, nor does it imply the need to achieve a single ideal of humanity. Rather, the mandate for honesty requires that one be who one really is, "good" and "bad," without duplicity or play-acting. Ideally, the patient will be freed to be who he really is and start growing into it as well.

Historically and in the current time, much of abuse involves the sexual exploitation of women by men. I think this puts male people, and male doctors in particular, in a very uncomfortable position vis-à-vis female clients with trauma histories. This merits discussion. Men with empathic powers may be horrified to learn of the damages women have suffered at the hands of other men; and they may feel ashamed, embarrassed, or guilty. Men whose powers tend to the technical may have trouble understanding how the emotional realms of the past color the present. They may feel annoyed at the "baggage" carried by the patient, impatient at how it slows down the good they can do, or suspicious that the patient may accuse them of something. Men who are young or inexperienced at their craft may be overwhelmed at the magnitude of the issues and hope that perhaps someone else can take care of it. Men who have had their own traumas (military, sexual, sexual orientation, familial, racial) may be ambivalent about the powers they really do possess as a clinician and feel reluctant to fully employ them. Conversely, they may be overly eager to display their power in professional situations, to no good end.

To all clinicians, I would say that the challenge of the work with the trauma survivor constitutes the challenge to know yourself, and to get out of the patient's way. Honesty here includes familiarity with yourself. If you know and can harness your reactions to your own past traumas, you can distinguish your experiences from your patient's. If you cannot, you run the risk of further burdening your already taxed patient. At best, your personal revelations and slant are of little use to your patient. At worst, this behavior is experienced as disempowering or re-traumatizing. I illustrate with two stories, the first from a related but non-medical setting.

> Eleven-year-old Sandra was engrossed in the shelves of the children's section of her local library, when a man who had followed her there came up next to her, unzipped his pants, displayed his full erection to her shocked face, and stared unrelentingly into her eyes. As quickly as she could, she gathered up her things, ran out of the library, and called her mother. The man vanished before the librarians could call the police. Sobbing, trembling, and inconsolable, Sandra went home with her

mom. Later that evening the police called, asking if she would come to headquarters to "look at some pictures and try to help us find him." Sandra went (with her mother). They showed her several unflattering mug shots of different men. Sandra knew they were just pictures but was repulsed by them, doing her best to compare them to her memory, and again began shaking. At the end of this, one of the policemen looked at her with a completely straight face and said, "You know, these guys are basically harmless."

The policeman was speaking from his own reality. To his knowledge and from his own experience, it was rare for a man with this type of perversion to physically harm or sexually assault a child. In addition, he was probably trying to comfort the girl, perhaps to help her get to sleep that night thinking she was "safe." But "unharmed" was not how she felt. "Unharmed" was not how she now was. She had just experienced an appalling life event from which she had to begin to recover.

Nicole was meeting her new primary care doctor for the first time. He was a middle-aged man with an excellent reputation and a successful practice who lived his entire life with a disfiguring physical disability. Nicole had done quite a lot of work on herself in therapy over the years. Once the medical history was taken, she decided it was important for their future relationship to disclose her past treatment by another physician, who had sexually assaulted her. The doctor listened to her somewhat halting, brief story, then said quickly and authoritatively, "Nicole, don't be a victim." Nicole was quite put off by this response. Her new doctor did not notice this. Nicole had not been seeking sympathy, nor advice on how to live. She had figured this man knew what it was to overcome life's misfortunes, and that her additional revelation would help them both form their new relationship based on truth. Now, she was getting an admonition she had not sought, and, perhaps, an implied judgment. She heard his fervent tone of voice, and realized he was urging on her *his own* life credo. The subject had triggered him. After a period of time, she left his practice. She had no desire to talk to this physician about what his words had done, or how she saw him. She saved that for her next doctor, who "just" listened, then thanked her for letting her know the whole story.

The need for respect bears emphasis. We've been taught since childhood to respect our elders, "do unto others," and so on. Professional schooling emphasizes the need to respect a patient's dignity. What's different in the situation with a trauma survivor is the profound *lack* of respect they have been afforded, often over a long period of time. This inevitably erodes aspects of their self-confidence and often their presentation of themselves. They may appear shabby, unwashed, naïve, inarticulate, unschooled. They may on the other hand be touchy, angry, or provocative. All outcomes are challenging to the clinician.

Implied here is the need to respect the magnitude of what this person has been through. Neglect and trauma, just like love and protection, are powerful forces. They have shaped your patient, and your job in dealing with them is not small.

Trust-building involves a commitment to keeping one's promises. This can involve small and large matters. If you say you will call, call. If you agree not to do a rectal exam, don't. If you have to change tack, discuss it ahead of time.

Finally, trust-building involves repair. All of us are imperfect. Many of us would like to be a lot better than we are. Some of us develop ego structures that see ourselves as better than we are. Others of us try hard to be "ideal" and then are overly hard on ourselves when we are not. We are all going to fail at knowing ourselves, appreciating the past, and being reliable. This is often felt acutely by survivors, whose abusers were duplicitous, seeking their own ends, and ruthless. What we can do differently is listen to our patients when they react, notice their body language and behavior, admit our shortcomings, and, when we err (as we all will), apologize. Many of these situations involve our own reactions to the needs of patients. We don't have to share that, as it may feel like blame or burden to a survivor. But we can acknowledge that our difficulty led us to make a mistake, and that we sense it might have been hard for the patient to bear. It can be humbling, but instructive, to be watched so closely by an expert (our patient) on power and powerlessness and given feedback we would perhaps rather not hear. This does not mean abasing ourselves in front of patients, but taking in the information, acknowledging it, and reflecting on it, both with patients and with trusted advisors of our own. It's a great way to learn. Meanwhile, our patients learn that not everyone in power is either perfect (which they often hope for) or abusive—but merely human. The fallibility of the trusted "other" is something survivors must work hard to accept. Doing so is one of the many difficult tasks of healing from trauma, and our errors are a part of our patients' growth when properly handled.

It can be helpful to remember, too, that we are seeing the *survivors* of past crimes, and battles. We aren't seeing the ones who had their lives taken away. Our patients may be critical, silent, angry, or wary, but they all have some measure of resilience. Usually, our mistakes will not kill them.

Empowerment

Some survivors of childhood trauma and violence seek out psychotherapy. Many can't, don't want to, or obtain limited results. Medical providers see survivors of all stripes. It's important to know that a medical relationship can be an important place for healing, and to know that it can also be useless to that end or even damaging.

We can adapt some knowledge from Judith Herman's now classic work, written for therapists:

> The first principle of recovery is the empowerment of the survivor. She must be the author and arbiter of her own recovery. Others may offer advice, support, assistance, affection, and care, but not cure. Many benevolent and well-intentioned attempts to assist the survivor founder because this fundamental principle of empowerment is not observed. No intervention that takes power away from the survivor can possibly foster her recovery, no matter how much it appears to be in her immediate best interest (4).

She goes on to caution that a patient who is suicidal, self-destructive, or harmful to others obviously must be deterred, with which I, of course, concur. But there is overall an inherent dilemma: How can we use a relationship, in which we as providers have so much power, as a source of power for a patient?

An initial step that must be taken is acknowledgment. This doctor–patient relationship is lopsided; providers really do have the powers that patients may perceive or react to. Our challenge is an ethical one: to use our powers for the benefit of others, to put the patient first. But it is also one of truth-telling, openness with our patients.

Second, we need some how-to. It's not so clear how we might foster the development of power in anyone. Edvin Schei has developed the idea of clinical leadership as a component of the use of power:

> Clinical leadership is a relational competence, where empathic perceptiveness and creativity render doctors capable of using their personal qualities, together with the scientific and technologic tools of medicine, to provide individualized help attuned to the particular circumstances of the patient. . . . The important point is to highlight that physicians have power in other people's lives and must develop adequate theoretical insights, skills, and character traits to wield that power for the benefit of their patients (5).

Favoring leadership over authority, Schei states that it is "more demanding . . . less predictable, and more prone to failure. . . . The notion of leadership does not entail that doctors should set the goals; rather, it suggests a facilitating role in the patient's attempts to understand and act wisely in times of crisis." He stresses the role of empathic dialogue between doctor and patient, and the need for "skillful improvisation" on the part of the clinician.

Here, the further development of the concept of servant-leadership may be relevant. Elements of this were laid out by Robert Greenleaf in his book of the same name in 1977. A businessman who studied, trained, and thought about effective leadership throughout his lifetime, Greenleaf came to embrace the following:

> *The great leader is seen as servant first. . . .* A new moral principle is emerging which holds that the only authority deserving one's allegiance is that which is freely and knowingly granted by the led to the leader in response to, and in proportion to, the clearly evident servant stature of the leader. Those who choose to follow this principle will not casually accept the authority of existing institutions. *Rather, they will freely respond only to individuals who are chosen as leaders because they are proven and trusted as servants.* (italics in original) (6)

The service mentioned here is that of the leader to the led. Its relevance to the use of power by the doctor for his patient I hope is obvious. Our job, then, is to believe in and recognize the strengths in our patients, to help them build on them, to partner with them in seeking control, and to learn that each person has his own source of authority, meaning, and power, waiting to be discovered when the two, doctor and patient, are ready. The task of the doctor is to believe that the patient can and must decide what is best for himself at any given time. The doctor has knowledge, experience, and tools. She is in charge of all of those. She is in charge of her own words and her awareness of their power. But the patient alone can decide what is best for him. The decision may appear arbitrary, odd, idiosyncratic, or contradictory. It may be at odds with "known medical truths." Often the doctor will go along unwillingly, or be tempted to scoff at the patient's "poor judgment." At these times it is important to remember that medical science can lead us to actions which are invasive, painful, biased, and motivated by unseen forces and one-sided truths—just as a patient's abuse was. Such a patient can help us take a second look at all our processes. And he can let us know when he is ready to proceed, despite the inevitability of flaws in the process.

Power and the Human Tangle of Oppression

I have mentioned in other chapters the victim/perpetrator/rescuer roles. Survivors can be damaged enough by childhood abuse that normal maturation and development is thwarted, and they instead "freeze" in their role, frequently as "victim." Living life as a victim invites others in proximity to join the drama as rescuers or, sometimes, perpetrators. Once operating within this triangle—or "quadrangle" if we add bystanders who avoid getting involved—players can and do shift roles, with the victim becoming a perpetrator, the rescuer a victim, and so on. It's a role-play in which everyone loses. If no one assumes a different approach, the whole system continues, and the original victims remain victims—unaware of their powers, not growing, dependent on others.

Health care providers can be ensnared in this cycle—as altruists, as people with tools and means, and simply as gullible, naïve, yet caring people. But if we become rescuers (or perpetrators or bystanders) then someone has to be the victim; and if we want to BE rescuers too much, we may end up ensuring that our patients remain victims in order to preserve the status quo—the geometric drama figure.

A reflection by Laura Chico, an American aid worker in post-genocide Rwanda, gives us food for thought. After discussing the dynamic above, she talks about how conflicted she felt after her arrival in the country, trying to decide how much and when to give, while being consistently asked for things from people who had very little: "Sometimes, problems are so fundamentally overwhelming that the only thing a new counselor knows to do is to give money or advice, trying to 'rescue' the person who is hurt rather than supporting, loving and guiding that person towards a solution." While not at all denying the need for material aid, on either a personal, institutional, or governmental level, she saw NGOs and others sucked into defining the terms and structures of recovery, sapping the strength, confidence, and native intelligence of the Rwandans. "The short-term benefits are great—the rescuers feel good about themselves and proud of the work and how much they have helped an organization or a person grow. The victims feel powerful—they have been able to get the most out of their donors.... They succeed in getting some money—but weaken their core. And both, trapped in this system which needs all three roles to sustain itself, take turns as the abuser, ensuring that the victims stay staunchly in their place."

Chico contrasts this with the action of a Rwandan woman, ultimately a colleague, whom she encountered in a healing community. This woman, now an adult striving to put her community back together, had at age 13 survived the invasion of her home by the opposing tribe, witnessing the contemporaneous murder of both parents, and had escaped death herself only by the humanity left in both her community *and* in her family's attackers. Following the genocide, she was approached by an ex-inmate who had been part of the marauding group which had killed her parents. He had served considerable time in his country's prison system and was now trying to start his life over. Despite fear, she listened as this man entrusted her with his own story of loss and exile. She realized that his trust was a rare gift. Then, she tried to work with his needs. "Here, the roles are becoming blurred—is (this Rwandan woman) a victim, or is she a rescuer? Is the man an abuser or victim? There is no clear path for untangling the corrosive and deeply ingrained roles of victims, rescuers and abusers. . . . It strikes me that (this woman) did not try to save this man, and he did not try to save her. Instead they have subtly reoriented themselves so that now they are side by side, looking at their broken lives, looking at their broken country, together. They are each on a journey, and for a while they fell in step with each other." (6).

If we can see ourselves more as listeners and companions, with the power to serve "side by side" with those who have suffered trauma in the past, we may be on the way to a fruitful partnership.

What Gets Learned

Faced with abusive power, children learn not only fear, self-loathing, and confusion, but also adaptive skills: the ability to dissociate (see Chapter 4); the ability to "read" their abuser (and others), to know his moods, his preferences, his weaknesses, his exploitability. They toughen and "grow up" too quickly, and make plans, which they may often carry out, to leave the situations they are in as soon as their means allow.

Such life experiences, however, will always travel with an abuse survivor. When he next encounters a situation involving personal powerlessness, his old knowledge may be called into play. In the medical encounter, the specters of illness, loss, and vulnerability, or even just getting undressed, can trigger such a scenario in the survivor's mind and then get played out in the experience of the provider and patient together.

Some survivors may respond to perceived powerlessness by bolting; others by "checking out," others by defiance (including defiance of one's own fear); others by developing such a haze of confusion and unreality that being with them feels like being in a dream; others by trying to seize control of some aspect of a situation. Underneath all of it is fear, and the memories of having been alone with a destructive force, faced with the worst that people can do. These are memories that few among us want to resurrect or imagine happening to ourselves.

Val

Val arrived at the door of our practice as a relatively young woman years ago and had seen a succession of providers. We knew from her answers on a written questionnaire that she came from another region of the country, and from a complex family. Both parents had died by the time we met her. She had broken several bones as a child, some requiring surgery or hospital stays. She was estranged from her entire family. Her answers on a mood questionnaire fulfilled the criteria for major depression. She had worked in a variety of jobs for some years, losing some of them because of "my temper." Eventually, she found satisfaction in working with children with emotional needs and ultimately got some education in this field. She lived alone.

After presenting this history, the practice did not see her for a year or two, as she made and did not keep three appointments. She came once for what was probably an acute gastroenteritis but allowed no physical exam. Several months later, she asked the receptionist to arrange for an EEG and told her that she had PTSD and didn't want anyone touching her.

Here is a good example of an initial negotiation around power. The patient is quite open on paper about some suggestive history, including major depression. Yet in the initial stages of this relationship, she has opted out of allowing her doctor one of his fundamental tools—the ability to examine her body. In fact, she often heralds her presence with a place on the appointment list but then fails to allow a sighting of her person at all. Val writes to me:

> Fear alone keeps Val from even making an appointment. To push through that and make the appointment is progress (the intent at that moment is to go.) When the time comes, the shame and fear . . . is overwhelming . . . The questions race. What to say? What is safe to say? What will happen? How to present?

This can be a challenging stage of a primary care relationship. For some, it will end before it really begins. Either the patient or the doctor will not tolerate the ambivalence involved. The patient may be overcome with fear and disappear. A provider must deal with annoyance or anger at an empty, "wasted" place on the appointment schedule. How does this patient's erratic behavior impact his day-to-day flow? When she does come, can he probe the behavior without judgment? Can he be ready for her, with openness and without retribution? She has told him enough that he should know this isn't easy for her, either.

Ultimately, Val did come back and allow a physical exam, done by a fourth-year medical student in the office. "Here for a full physical for medication change . . . no complaints," stated the student. Val's medications, (which now included some antidepressants) and a weight gain were both recorded, but no other history appears. A full physical, including a scantily described pelvic exam, was done. There was no evidence of deductive reasoning at the end of the student's note: "39 yo WF w psychiatric hx-depression here for physical exam" was the conclusion. It is difficult to know what really transpired here. One can certainly understand a student's inability to comprehend what she was getting into. One might wonder what kind of state both she and the patient were in. Certainly, the notes taken by the student appear to lack meaning and connection. Here is another danger of treating the "hiding" patient, the one who presents only carefully selected parts of herself. The danger is that you are tempted to be present only in part yourself. Val writes:

> Partly there? No! All is present. Every step, every moment is measured. Taken carefully and fearfully, she is allowing somebody to interact with her body.
>
> She has <u>no</u> positive experiences with this.

Guardedness and questions about trustworthiness are foremost. Did the student sense this? In *Confronting Chronic Neglect*, the Institute of Medicine's 2002 report on violence education, medical educators are encouraged to help trainees learn to deal with the effects of family violence on their patients (and themselves) (8). Like many other students, this one was progressing through her education without any such mentoring. Such an absence, I believe, contributed to the lack of vitality in this encounter.

The doctor who founded the practice retired, the medical student he had overseen moved on, and over the next five years, Val saw two other primary care doctors at the practice who came and ultimately left. With each, she consented to examinations and revealed a bit more about herself. The rudiments of a sexual history emerged. This gave rise to no current concerns, as she had been celibate for years. She remained morbidly obese. She had had a remote period of alcoholic drinking. She was now under the care of a psychiatrist, who was seeing her for a greatly reduced fee and was working with her on a complex medication regime. This psychiatrist stressed the importance of regular medical care. Val now usually came to her appointments, which were scheduled around the demands of her job. She allowed blood work. She agreed to mammograms during appointments, but never did them. When abnormal liver tests worried her psychiatrist, she once allowed a liver ultrasound, showing only fatty liver. She mostly refused to do any more evaluation, except to have her blood monitored, even when her mood darkened or her liver looked worse. Her psychiatrist became the patient's medical advocate, calling with concerns and pleading, at times successfully, with the patient to have evaluations done.

I had come to the practice during this same five-year period, after the founder left. Val's psychiatrist called me, as one of the few remaining clinicians at the practice after the coming-and-going of now three doctors. The psychiatrist outlined Val's trauma history, still unknown to any of her prior providers, and her need for a stable figure. The psychiatrist had concerns about lab work, including liver tests and an abnormal blood sugar, especially in the context of multiple powerful medications. The patient did not call. The psychiatrist and I agreed on a monitoring interval, with which Val complied, but she did not return to actually see any of the doctors for another year and a half.

It cannot have been easy for Val to have this succession of medical practitioners. Nevertheless, she trusted us to the extent that we were her source for health care when needed; we monitored her to the extent that she allowed, and perhaps most importantly, there was a progressive sharing of intimate information, slowly over the years. These might all be seen as signs of progress, or stability within instability. It was her psychiatrist whom she really seemed to trust.

She came for a full exam (meeting me for the first time) some years ago: "Val states that she is here only because her psychiatrist 'would shoot me if I didn't come' ". Val said this with both a straight face and with the slightest hint of humor—a mature, battle-hardened human being. She was trying to start a more active lifestyle. She was still taking numerous psychiatric medications. She told me that her father, who had left her family about five years before, had died of AIDS, and that he had lived a closeted gay lifestyle before he left the family and came out.

"She states that she gets physical exams somewhat under duress, that she 'doesn't like being touched,' has never gotten a mammogram for this reason, and 'spaces out' to cope with physical exams." Periods were still regular. She was 48. She hadn't been sexually active in years but had had a boyfriend many years ago. She remained very overweight at 228 pounds, 61 inches. I wrote that she was "terse but cooperative." She smelled unwashed. She was hypertensive. She had lost all her upper teeth, and teeth that were left were in poor shape. She had fungal infection between her toes. She agreed to blood work and discussed having a mammogram. She agreed to taking a requisition for it, both of us having discussed that having it was a reminder of my hope she would do it. She refused a tetanus booster.

So here we have Val openly telling me that I can get her to water but can't make her drink. She will allow a physical exam, but she doesn't have to 'be there' (dissociation). Val writes:

> No, you can't force me to drink. But you can walk alongside up to the next hurdle/challenge. Allow the time needed to figure out how to get over. (What are the dangers? What are the pros? All have to be weighed first.) Patience . . . Any open

> sharing of personal information had an extreme cost. It broke all the rules, instilled terror of retaliation. But took the chance and shared.

Her lack of bathing, dental care, and foot care were further evidence of her distancing others, as well as distance from her own body. There was no truculence in her tone; she was honestly providing me with information about herself.

How might I understand her position? What power did I have to convince her to allow me to help her help herself? I felt that information ("skin is healthier if you bathe"), shaming ("you have an odor"), and intimidation ("you are at higher than average risk for breast cancer, you should be having mammograms") would be of no use. All seemed counterproductive. Val had to submit to shame and fear in the past; she will do so no longer. Living completely inside of her body may be too dangerous at present. Touch is likely a reminder not only that she actually exists, but that touch and existence were corrupted for her in some unspeakable way. Despite years of psychiatric treatment, these issues are not faceable at this moment. We have to work around them. We will have to look for ways to empower her to "touch" her own existence, her own body—at her own speed. Val again:

> You cannot give "power"—people who have come through traumas bring with them rules and actions that are engraved in stone on the soul of the individual. You need to help them feel they can x or cannot y without loss of life. Without retribution. It's to assist in the overcoming of the feeling of terror, of extreme dread that arises when told just go ahead and do x—the hell, you say . . . There is lots of power but none
>
> of it belongs to the person, and it all belongs to the past. You want to help—walk with me through the many "blocks" in my psyche. Go
>
> through the "You're not allowed to's," the "If you do then I will hurt you's," the "there is no laughing, no crying" rules, the "you own nothing here," the "you don't exist" messages, the "you have to be alone" messages—"there will be no friends, no one comes here; you can't associate with them."

Blood work revealed a few days later that she was now mildly diabetic and still had hyperlipidemia. According to current guidelines, she would need several new medications. My heart sank. Would she ever agree to do anything? I wrote her, telling her that "Yikes! I have to see you again!" and suggesting she check her own blood pressure for a while before she came. In doing so, I hoped to reach the Val who had a fledgling sense of irony—which is, after all, the ability to step outside one's current troubles, see them in perspective, and compare them perhaps to some element of human history. This ability to be both in and out of a negative experience is a crucial first step in the recovery from PTSD (see Chapter 3), and one I hoped she would be able to do. ("I'm only here because my therapist would kill me . . .") In addition, by suggesting she take her own blood pressure, I hoped to hand over control in managing her disease.

Much to my surprise and delight, she showed up two months later. We talked about the "metabolic syndrome," the role of weight loss, exercise, diet, and so on. There was a family history of diabetes in her brother; she didn't know about her father. She hadn't taken her blood pressure or bought a cuff. She stated that at the human service center where she was currently working, there **was** no blood pressure cuff. She was strategizing about weight loss with her therapist. She agreed to start an ACE inhibitor and to check a glycohemoglobin. Fortunately, the latter was in the realm of "good control" and no diabetes medication per se had to be begun.

One month later, she returned to check on the blood pressure. She had purchased a wrist cuff – cheaper, touching only a small surface of her arm. Her measurements showed improvement, and in the office, using the appropriate cuff for her arm, her blood pressure was now normal. Despite a weight gain of nine pounds, I told her she had achieved "success" and should go away for three months and not see me at all. She was quite happy with that. I chose not to talk about weight, lifestyle, cholesterol drugs, or anything else I was "supposed" to. I wanted her to feel free of all of this for some time and to have a simple, indubitable, and reasonably painless success.

We were at a beginning. We had begun working with small, tolerable building blocks. A great deal of medication, and a long, carefully built psychiatric relationship had preceded our work together. In negotiating the new challenges, I tried to sense where her strengths lay, to work with and within her defenses, and to be her companion in surveying her (and our) "Rwanda"—the damaged but improving and improvable landscape of her body and soul to which her life had led her, thus far.

Other Negotiations

Some adult survivors take their need for power in a direction different than Val did. Instead of disappearing, they challenge us as providers and challenge our systems of care. They may particularly challenge the parts of us that feel we need fairly absolute power over something—our telephone hours, our schedules, our reputations, our authority. Usually, these challenges inconveniently display to us and perhaps others how our functions and dysfunctions are intimately woven together. These can be hateful, difficult patients. When all is said and done, they have much to teach us about what we are really good for, and how to have faith in ourselves despite our imperfections. Ultimately, this is a lesson that such patients need to learn as well. The people entrusted to take care of them as children failed miserably and did terrible damage. Now, as adults, these clients have to learn to trust people who have their interest at heart but who will still fail, sometimes. Despite their best efforts, we are truly needed, at times.

The story of Elora in Chapter 3 can be read as that of such a patient. Like Val, Elora had initially refused a physical exam by a doctor she did not know or trust. Unlike her, she told her new doctor what she needed and from whom she wanted it (a tubal ligation), implying that the doctor was (as the "gatekeeper") simply a means to an end.

Things got more complicated and difficult with the onset of the thoracic outlet symptoms. Elora knew she needed help. I knew that I was unfamiliar with her presentation, but also that I was uneasy and worried about it. The person available to help us as a consultant was not someone with the ideal personality to deal with someone for whom control and power were important, because he had his own issues with them (in my opinion). Nevertheless, time seemed of the essence.

The surgeon was annoyed at what seemed to him to be an unnecessary interruption of his routine. Moreover, this surgeon felt I had blown things out of proportion—"the patient is referred here today for 'lack of pulses.'" In retrospect, he arrived at a premature closure with the patient, sending her to another specialist who ultimately proved to be irrelevant. The patient interpreted this second referral as belittling and concluded that the vascular surgeon was incompetent in return. When she changed vascular surgeons, Elora made no bones to their office staff about her opinion of the first surgeon, particularly when the diagnosis was ultimately made under rushed circumstances, requiring emergency surgery to save her arm. This offended the first surgeon greatly.

Before her diagnosis was made, during the period of uncertainty and alarm, Elora responded by hounding my office, bullying the staff, and generally bludgeoning her way to the top of the pile. She needed attention, and this is how she got it. Similarly, when both her surgeons and I initially missed her hemothorax, several months later she responded with understandable agitation and demands, vigorously, and eventually got what she needed.

What enabled our relationship to stand up to failure and what must have felt again like abandonment of her needs, when others had not? First, we all (due to Elora's persistence) got lucky—and her function and body were saved. For this I am forever grateful (as is she). Elora had survived in her life by not being willing to take a place in line. She survived (unlike Val) by tuning into her own body. She survived by being scathing when things weren't going well. She was "not a nice patient."

Second, there is need for humility in the practice of medicine. Though we as medical professionals are charged with care of people's health, and though medicine has made great strides in the last century and current decades, still, what we do not know outweighs what we do. This is especially true in the area of somatic symptoms without known cause (see Chapter 7). As we all know, these symptoms dangerously overlap with "what we do know but have not yet figured out." In addition, success in diagnosis and treatment is often built on the empiric trial and error of those who come before us. Acknowledgment is only fair.

Finally, honesty again helps. It's best to be transparent about what we do and don't know, and what we can and can't yet do.

Most germane to this chapter, however, are the lessons about power in the care of all patients, especially adult survivors. These recap the themes discussed earlier: those of trust, empowerment, and victimization and its perpetuation. The establishment of trust between doctor and patient, once present, places an enormous positive burden on the provider to respond, to do what is needed. In primary care, this translates to advocacy, reflection, and "presence." Being a "leader" or "servant leader," or "honest companion" of such a patient mandates a position of subtle oscillation between listening and steering the boat together. When the victim/patient acts like a perpetrator, or seems to, one must, as provider, not step into the emotional position of victim, rescuer, or passive bystander but maintain the ability to either shift roles, or often to respectfully take control until the patient has regained it. The provider can also choose to remain outside of the quadrangle entirely, aware of dynamics but in some important way unmoved, and wait without judgment for the storm to subside. Elora's ultimate surgeon stood up for his colleague (whom Elora denigrated) and proceeded on facts and findings. He did not elevate himself as her hero. I tried to remind myself, and the patient, that we were in uncharted waters, doing the best we could. There was and would be no perfection here. We all muddled through it, somehow.

References

1. From *Care of the Soul*, by Thomas Moore. Copyright © 1992 by Thomas Moore. Used by permission of HarperCollins Publishers. Also Reproduced with permission of Licensor through PLS Clear, 1992.
2. Davies JM and Frawley MG, *Treating the Adult Survivor of Childhood Sexual Abuse: A Psychoanalytic Perspective*, pp. 105–106, Basic Books, 1994.
3. Brownmiller S, *Against Our Will: Men, Women, and Rape*, p. 116, Ballantine Books, Random House, 1975.

4. Herman J, *Trauma and Recovery*, p. 133, Basic Books, Harper Collins Publishers, 1992.
5. Schei E, "Doctoring as leadership: the power to heal," *Perspectives in Biology and Medicine* 49(3): 393–406, 2006.
6. Chico LS, "Frozen in time: escaping the victim-abuser-rescuer triangle," PeaceWays, African Great Lakes Initiative of the Friends Peace Teams I, 2, Fall 2006.
7. Greenleaf RK, *Servant Leadership: A Journey into the Nature of Legitimate Power and Greatness*, Paulist Press, 1977.
8. Cohn F, Salmon ME, and Stobo JD (eds.), *Confronting Chronic Neglect, The Education and Training of Health Professionals on Family Violence*, National Academy Press, Washington, DC, 2002.

6

Self-Harm

Nothing has changed.
Except for the courses of rivers,
the contours of forests, seashores, deserts, and icebergs.
Among these landscapes the poor soul winds,
vanishes, returns, approaches, recedes.
A stranger to itself, evasive,
at one moment sure, the next unsure of its existence,
while the body is and is and is
and has no place to go (1).

Introduction

People in medicine have trouble, sometimes, with patients who exhibit self-destructive behavior. For instance, until the middle of the last century, alcoholism was understood to be a vice. It produced antisocial conduct and/or indicated a character weakness. During the last six or seven decades, it has come to be labeled and understood as a "disease." It is a disease that has physical, social, and spiritual manifestations, and its treatment, for the most part, is social (2). The "disease" label superficially removes our previous judgments. Our "disease understanding" does not make it any easier to cope with the despair we feel when a cirrhotic relapses with hepatitis, or when we must recycle a young person, again, through detox. Similarly, feelings of anger at the drug-seeker trying to manipulate us or our systems, the frustration and terror of dealing with a young anorexic, the worry or panic when a teenager begins to cut herself, are all difficult to bear. Such feelings easily channel themselves into judgments, passive-aggressive behavior, and unhelpful acts on the part of would-be "helpers."

Reece (3) writes:

> Accident and Emergency departments are concerned with trauma whatever the source or client age. This mixed trauma culture can be a distressing place, not least

for women whose self-injury is "self-inflicted" rather than accidental in nature. The women, who might be survivors of childhood sexual abuse, are sometimes viewed as service abusers, on occasions subjected to misinterpretation, labeled as "timewasters" and consequently stigmatized.

Understanding Stigma

In preparing to deal with clients who have histories of childhood abuse, we must look through such initial reactions and become ready to deal with laden souls. We must learn to channel our own reactions and to get into a constructive position with patients. It is difficult to know how to be helpful, particularly when burdened with our own feelings. Eating disorders and addiction are illnesses not so easy to treat. They are some of the most prevalent, harmful, and resistant disorders in our culture today. We are taught little about them during training, and when we move into practice we don't find many tested drugs or methods we can utilize for our patients. We simply don't know what to do and are not comfortable with how to be.

Injury and Injury to the Self

The topics for this chapter will include addiction, self-mutilation, and death. Eating disorders will be visited. We will discuss addiction to and unsafe use of alcohol and prescription drugs. We'll examine taking up arms against oneself, self-burning, cutting, and sudden death.

Of course, not all addicts have histories of abuse. Nor do any of these behaviors have a single cause. They all appear to have multiple roots in genetics, environment, personal history, family history, culture, availability of lethal agents, and so on. In a textbook with another title, I don't believe these conditions would be in the same chapter.

I am grouping them in this chapter because people with abuse histories, more commonly than those without such histories, choose to hurt themselves—"choice" being perhaps an inaccurate term. The fact that they do so is one of the subjects of this chapter; responses engendered in health care providers is another. In addition, I hope that examining the links between past abuse and current self-harm, including detailed study of a few patients' stories, will help us all understand what we can and should do, and what not to do. We will look at what some of the pitfalls for patients and their caregivers may be.

All self-injurious behaviors have some definable causes. However, interestingly, once they have taken hold they seem to be capable, like some invasive species, of developing a life and trajectory all their own. They appear to exist on their own; they obey certain laws of their own, and they can continue, independently, to do damage to a patient's body, mind, and spirit. For instance, alcohol, used in a vulnerable person to bolster self-esteem or assuage negative feelings, often results in addiction, and repeated use can cause liver, myocardial, and nervous system damage. Bulimia can lead to disordered gastrointestinal function, dental decay, and severe electrolyte disturbances, as well as social degeneration. Once rooted, these diseases may appear both to their sufferers and their providers to be "the illness." They ARE diseases to treat. Alcoholism and drug addiction treatment must often precede or parallel effective treatment for PTSD and other disorders of trauma. However, treatment of the whole human is not complete, and is less likely be successful longitudinally, without an exploration of what led the person to the self-destructive behavior in the first place. Primary care and other providers owe it to themselves and their patients to gain, hold, and explore this knowledge with their patients in a setting safe for both.

Felitti (4), working in the preventive health domain, has with others been carrying out long-term studies of the effects of "adverse childhood experiences" (ACEs) on many aspects of adult health. In his words:

> Many of our most intractable public health problems are the result of compensatory behaviors like smoking, overeating, and alcohol and drug use, which provide immediate partial relief from the emotional problems caused by traumatic childhood experiences. Those experiences are generally unrecognized and become lost in time, where they are protected by shame, by secrecy, and by social taboos against exploring certain areas of human experience. A public health paradox becomes apparent wherein the public health *problem* is also often an unconsciously attempted *solution* (italics his). Not surprisingly, it is hard to give up something that almost works, particularly at the behest of someone who issues cautionary advice without any idea of what is really going on. For instance, in the public health onslaught against smoking, we have lost sight of the psychoactive benefits of nicotine, which is well documented as having antianxiety, antidepressant, anger suppressant, and appetite suppressant properties.

Felitti and his co-researcher Anda appeared some years ago on National Public Radio (5) in an eight-minute segment as part of a series on "What Shapes Health." He was discussing the "ACE score" (6) a simple rubric he devised for clinicians to use to begin an exploration of their patients' exposure as children to traumatic experiences, including abuse, neglect, death, or incarceration of a parent. Felitti and his co-researchers have documented the positive correlation between the number of ACEs and negative health outcomes, including alcoholism, coronary artery disease, addiction, depression, and suicide (7). The segment highlighted the failure of this little test to be used widely and speculated on reasons why.

Shortly thereafter, as part of a news feed online about the segment, the public was offered the question "what is your ACE score?" and the opportunity to take the brief test and "learn one's score" as if they were applying for a mortgage. Though increasing public awareness of the link between early experience and health is surely a good thing, I believe this type of publicity misses a good part of the point. The segment featured Fellitti and an actual patient discussing some of her positive ACE questions, with Fellitti (a retired primary care physician as well as researcher) modeling the kind of sympathetic, open-ended, non-judgmental and safe exploration with a patient that we could all hope to emulate. The patient later commented that as a result, she had begun to think about her childhood and her health in an entirely new way. Fellitti noted the healing role of this type of conversation, in which one person shares shameful or deeply distressing experiences with another, then "leaves with the understanding that they are still an acceptable member of the human race." The unburdening of negative feeling by the doctor and the patient together freed the patient to begin, perhaps, to work with herself in a new way. The segment admitted that the conversation took extra time—the visit was 30 minutes instead of 20. It left us to ponder the value added.

Why don't we ask?

There are the obvious answers: the answers take more time, that time is not reimbursed, we were not taught to do so, and so forth. All are true. The deeper reasons may be that we don't know what to do with the answers—and more, we don't know what to do with how we feel about the answers.

Cutting

Straker (8) has recently explored the possible meanings—to the patient and to the clinician—of acts of self-mutilation.

"[S]elf-cutting remains disturbing to most clinicians, who see its death-dealing aspects, as opposed to its more enlivening ones," says Straker. Like a suicidal gesture, self-cutting could be viewed as an echo, or a reminder of the possibility of a more lethal act. We all know the deadly progression of an addicted life, and the unheralded and catastrophic moves of suicidality.

By "enlivening," on the other hand, I understand Straker to mean offering a window into a genuine interpersonal exchange, or possibly "helping the patient to achieve greater clarity and control over her behavior, and greater freedom from the control the behavior has over herself."

I remember a moment during an initial physical exam of a middle-aged woman, years ago. After a lengthy and mutual-feeling history, she changed into a johnny. During the physical exam, I came upon her wrists and forearms, covered with multiple transverse straight scars, all healed, appearing to be old but of varying ages. None of this had come out in the history. I looked at the scars, then looked at her, she looked back at me, and there was a wholly new moment between us. She had begun to show me her "true" past. What did the scars say? They said, "There is a part of me I have not yet shared." They said, "I did this," and "I am someone who did this." They, and her silence until that moment, said, "I challenge you to even begin to understand."

So there can be fear and anxiety on our part; there can even be shame, perhaps, at not having known this before or not wanting to know. There can also be disgust, revulsion at the mess people can make of themselves. There can be impatience—at how much time this behavior takes, at how long it takes to give it up. Finally, there is fatigue. Getting to the root of all this is a long, arduous, and potentially unsuccessful project. We know we're not supposed to display any of these feelings to patients. Maybe we think we are not even supposed to have them. We also know people aren't supposed to do these things to themselves, or us. All of this leads us to become annoyed and dismissive: the grounds for judgment. Self-harmers appear to be hysterical attention-getters (see the Reece article quoted above); alcoholics weak, perhaps laughable and reprehensible problems; and suicidal people objects of pity.

Do we feel this way about a middle-aged man in the middle of an acute coronary syndrome? Coronary disease, after all, is one of the outcomes of a higher ACE score. This seems less likely, though the understanding of "coronary risk factors" has moved us minimally toward a comprehension of the role of behavior in that disease. It has probably not moved us toward understanding the determinants of that behavior. We can now put in a stent almost as easily as we can sew up a laceration or have a 30-minute conversation about ACEs. (These, of course, pay quite differently. In part, this discrepancy may reflect dominant cultural views regarding the "value" of the patient. It may also reflect how well hidden the diseases seem to be from their origins in childhood maltreatment.) How do we begin to understand and moderate the overeating, the survival in corporate culture, the relentless drive to the top, the lack of self-care, exercise, and moderation, and the nicotine addiction that led to the disease? We have similar—and similarly difficult—work with the cutter/addict/

harmer. The scar, and the ruptured plaque, are the signposts that point toward the work to be done.

One difference is that in putting in the stent or adhering to "evidence-based guidelines" for cholesterol treatment, we can feel that we are "doing something." We all want to know what we can DO when we recognize a problem. My answer for the treater of those who self-harm: we can listen deeply, learn more about the patient, work to keep him safer; create a setting that empowers the patient to work on her own problem; and offer our strength and our hope, continuing all the while to learn and acquire true wisdom. We can also try to remain honest, because we will make many mistakes, some of which will be shameful to us. We must always work on forgiving ourselves, too.

Linnea

We had over 20 years of medical records on Linnea when she first came to our practice, leaving her old doctor due to a change in health insurance. She'd had remote Bell's palsy, two home births, a few minor complaints. Eight years ago, she had developed intermittent peptic symptoms, both related and unrelated, it seemed, to h. pylori. These responded to treatment but recurred intermittently. Low back pain had been an issue. She was perimenopausal. She was married, and her two children were in late adolescence when we met her.

Months before, however, she had lost 20 pounds, unexpectedly, and saw her old doctor ". . . under a lot of stress, not eating. Psychologist wanted us to order many labs." A physical examination was normal, and lab work revealed only a mild leukopenia. Depression was mentioned in the chart for the first time. "She is eating minimally. She states that it is not really a lack of appetite but more that she just does not allow herself to eat. Probably it is part of a control issue." She was encouraged to follow up with a new primary care physician to "repeat her white blood cell count."

Linnaea came about three months later, first seeing the physician assistant, then me. She had been cutting her arms with a knife, and this was why she came, she said. Her left forearm showed 15 superficial lacerations in various states of healing. Her weight was stable. She had cut herself in the past but not for a long while, until the last few months. She was in psychotherapy and told us that she had "PTSD." The PA discussed parameters of safety with the patient, who agreed, and agreed to close follow-up. When I first saw Linnaea a week later, she told me she had begun to be bulimic again, mentioning that this was a problem for her in high school. In college, she became anorexic. Maximum weight loss had been about 20% of her body weight. She was currently at a BMI of 20 and admitted to some fanatic exercise. She didn't go into any details about her therapy and appeared reticent to discuss it.

"Because of unbearable feelings, she has for the past two months apparently scarified herself, particularly in her left upper extremity. She has never required stitches although a couple of them were fairly deep. The scarification 'is the only thing that reveals (? relieves) the feeling and brings me back to earth. Otherwise, I'm one here, one there.' She is sometimes aware of an odd feeling in her skin, as if a 'cold wind of cosmic despair is blowing on my back.' She relieves this by massage."

Review of systems revealed that she had had recurrent sinusitis, some asthma, and that "the last time she vomited was about six months ago because she 'felt disgusting.' Bowels are entirely regular. Her sex life is fine." Her physical exam revealed a woman who appeared thin, intelligent, and younger than her stated age. It showed the scars, the residual Bell's palsy, a stable (low) weight, and was otherwise ok.

Many concerns here confront the practitioner. The weight loss, given the above history, appears explained, though now we know she has an eating disorder. What will she need from us for that? For insurance reasons, she has had to start a new primary care relationship just as these other troubles are emerging. We don't know what the psychological issues are, and she is reluctant to name them but gives vivid descriptions of bits of her inner state. These are not symptoms we know how to treat, but she wants us to know about them. She has evidence of past and present self-harm. She appears almost childlike in her thinness, youthfulness, vulnerability. Yet there is something of the crone in the person who notices the "cold wind of cosmic despair blowing." Where does one start?

I made my first problem list for Linnea: (I quote, with current commentary in parentheses.)

1. Anorexia. Patient was told to contact me if her weight dropped close to 102 and that she should try, at a minimum, to hover above a baseline weight that was still healthy for her. She agrees to attempt this.
2. Self-mutilation. (I apparently had no thoughts about what to do about this.)
3. Emotional problems underlying all these, of unclear nature right now.
4. Lingering sinus inflammation.
5. Strong family history of cancer—plans for screening made. (I didn't include this in the above history.)
6. History of right Bell's palsy.
7. Asthma with exposure to cold air.

I note now that I did not mention specifically her "unbearable feelings," her "felt disgusting," nor her despair. I might now group them in #3 rather than putting "emotional problems" or her offered "PTSD." The PTSD label may be her way of clueing us in to the presence of past trauma, whatever it was. If it is true, it hints at intrusive states of feeling out of control, feeling negative about oneself and others, feeling hopeless (see Chapter 3). But we don't really know what she means. It is important to realize that at least some self-harm in trauma patients arises from welling-up of such unbearable feelings and being unable to control them or one's actions.

From a trauma therapy group for women (8):

Participant 1: I never feel happy, just frustrated, or bored, Then, when I'm stressed, it gets really bad and I feel like I'm going crazy, like I just can't take it.

P2: Sometimes I feel at the end of my rope, too, but I have noticed that since I've been coming to these sessions, I've felt happy once in a while. It never lasts, though.

P3: You have to have something to feel happy about before you're gonna feel happy. I feel lonely most of the time because people don't want to be around me. I'm a downer.

In response to a question from the group leader about what feeling out of control feels like:

P1: What are you talking about, it feels like being out of control, crazy, you know . . . My whole body changes, I feel hot and tingly all over.

P2: I know what you mean. I'm like a volcano that is just ready to blow.

P3: For me, it's like an energy rush. Everything inside is racing at maximum speed. I can't slow down, but it's all on the inside.

P1: I can relate. I'm exploding inside. I just have to punch something or cut myself.

P4: I'm just the opposite. When I'm out of control, I just shut down. I go on remote.

P5: For me, it's all about anger. I feel just full of rage and I know if I had a gun or something, I would just want to blow somebody's head off . . . just whoever gets in my way. You better not be in my way when I'm like that.

In response to a question from the leader about what happens if you don't shut down, punch someone, or cut yourself?

P2: You don't want to know. She just gets so mad and hopeless that she'll take it out on somebody, or so depressed that she wants to kill herself. That's what I do if I can't let it out when I feel that worked up. Then, I don't feel anything anymore, like I empty my insides out.

P4: Yeah, I don't want anyone else to get hurt like I have. I'd rather just go away.

P5: I'll get revenge if they do me wrong. That makes me feel better. They deserve it. I don't go looking for trouble, but if you bring it to me, then we're going the whole distance (9).

Although it may be hard for a clinician to understand what leads patients to cut (for instance), these women all understand each other quickly. They know this feeling of inner agitation, as well as its sequelae—action, or dissociation—and they recognize it, however it is expressed in each other.

They all also seem to realize that this can be a dangerous state to be in; they feel dangerous to others and warn others to stay away. Women in this group take the alternative of taking it out on themselves rather than another, though the option of hurting others is definitely there. In this way, they are protecting the "other" from harm, in the way that they were NOT protected. In at least some self-harm, then, there may be a misguided but believable justice function at work. Cutting could be seen in this way as a form of strength on the part of the patient, an attempt to keep even healthy anger and violent feelings from hurting other people. It also may be an attempt to show, perhaps to their perpetrators, that there is, or was, another way.

Cutting takes place in the here and now, and it also has a communication function, like much of nonverbal human behavior. Straker (8) studied a group of middle-class therapy patients who were cutting themselves. She compares the "scar" to writing, to inscription, to naming and to characterizing. The body is a tablet upon which such writing can take place. We can understand that at the moment it occurs, self-harm may paradoxically render two-way communication impossible (drunkenness, overdose, suicide attempt, hemorrhage). But when the acute wounds heal, or after the episode ends, we, as guardians of the health of the physical bodies of persons, are privileged to be both the discoverers **and** the receivers of this sort of communication. In fact, it may have been directed toward us, as the healers of the human race, if we can ready ourselves to truly hear what is (not being) "said."

Straker, a psychologist, then analyzes what brings the cutter to cut. Her theme is that self-harmers experience "a felt disturbance in relation to language." Many of those whose stories she analyzed so closely were articulate, literate women. Yet when it came to the experiences leading to cutting, there were no words they could use to convey the emotions experienced that led them to cut. Implied here, I believe, were the childhood experiences of terror, rage, betrayal, and shame we have discussed before, carried with these people unfiltered and unprocessed into adulthood. Straker sees this failure of the development of language use in such patients as an outgrowth of the abuse itself; that it co-opted the ability to "use one's words."

There are some questions about language and abuse experiences here. Is it conceivable that there are human experiences that cannot be put into words? Is it possible that the nature of language prohibits certain experiences and feelings from linguistic communication? Second, is there something about some abuse experiences that are better communicated, or feel better communicated nonverbally? Third, is every destructive "inscription" on the body—suicide, drug addiction, cutting, necessarily communication to anyone other than the self? Conversely, since language conjures a give and take, does such self-abuse, done wordlessly, imply that there is someone (including, perhaps, us as health care professionals) who is not listening? Could it be that our society and institutions would just prefer not to hear?

Over the past several decades, there has been an explosion of research on brain development and function. Results from studies on subjects abused and neglected as children show a wide variety of structural abnormalities, including in the corpus callosum, hippocampus, and amygdala. Gray matter volume as a whole has been shown to be decreased in such subjects. Adults exposed to childhood parental verbal abuse show changes in the arcuate fasciculus (which connects Wernicke's and Broca's areas) and display lower verbal IQ scores (10). How all of this may tie in with language function, impulse control, and mood is only beginning to be sorted out. As discussed in previous chapters, brain anatomy and function seem demonstrably affected by adverse childhood experiences.

Thus, there is much in the act of cutting, and other acts against the self, to give us pause. I have tried to outline above how we might move from fear, annoyance, and derision to honor, perhaps; skillfulness, hopefully; and certainly receptivity. Of course, we hope to journey with the patient to other, less self-destructive forms of communication and justice-seeking. We can only do that if we listen, hear where it all comes from, and form an alliance that fosters the patient's moves toward health.

Linnea had some bouts with recurrent sinusitis, then returned about a year and a half later for a short visit "mostly to make sure I am healthy." I wrote: "Patient has continued with anorexia. She has continued to have severe inter psychic (sic) stress. She is only rarely bulimic, last was about 6 weeks ago. Usually, it is only one episode. She is just not eating much. In the summer, she was on retreat, ate less and thinks she got under 100 lbs. And probably has gained a little since then. She assures me that 'despite things looking worse on the outside, things on the inside are looking better.' She notes that her hair is falling out, her nails are chipping and that she experiences 'ripples' in her thighs. However, she remains physically active. Does not experience any dizziness or weakness, no loss of muscle power, no difficulty getting up stairs, etc." I noted that she was nonpostural and did not have a lot of alopecia; she had no discernible muscle weakness. "Her last cutting episode was about a month ago and she was seen in the ER and sutured without any questions asked."

"She also assures me that her sister who called is a very negative person and she does not wish any information released to her."

Later that month, Linnaea returned for a full exam: "The patient has been working hard in psychotherapy over the past year. She has recovered more memories of emotional, sexual and physical abuse by both parents. Patient was a middle child. Her older sister was also abused. Her younger was spared. The patient felt that she always knew these things, but somehow, they have become much more real. She has undergone a separation and divorce in the last 9 mos. She is currently living with her (teenaged) son.

"Her chief concerns are a feeling that occasionally her muscles are rippling particularly in her thighs. Over the summer when she was eating poorly, she also awoke at night with muscle cramps. Recent lab work was normal. She has lost even further weight over the summer but has regained some of it. Several weeks ago, she did have another incident of self-mutilation, deeper than before. 'I made a mess and I am not going to be doing it again.' " (This was said in new tone for her, that of an adult taking charge without harmful blaming). "She is increasingly aware that her wors(t) enemy is herself. 'I see myself in the mirror and I see my attacker.' " Exam was normal, (though she was thin at 106 pounds and 64 inches) save for the healed and healing (more recent, deeper) scars, and residual old Bell's palsy. Lab work ok. Muscle rippling unexplained.

Linnea felt healthier, despite her emaciation. Was she? On the one hand, there are signs of malnutrition, or severe stress—her nails, her weight, her hair. On the other hand, she was setting boundaries with her family (and me). She was (for now) cutting less. Linnea the "attentive, adult parent" was more inclined to put a stop to self-abuse. Finally, she was growing in her self-awareness, dramatically expressed ("I see myself in the mirror," etc.)

What about the muscles? Was Linnea describing fasciculations? I didn't see any, nor any weakness. Should she see a neurologist? Were the muscle cramps related to electrolyte disturbances while starving (possibly). Or could this be a body memory of sexual abuse, emerging along with the other things she "knew all along"? I elected to leave this complaint alone, and it never resurfaced.

Finally, I would note the destructive effect past abuse has on people's current most important relationships. Linnea cannot trust her sister (who may yet understand her). Linnea leaves her husband and marriage of many years, as her true self and history are emerging. There are chasms where there could have been intimacy but perhaps never was.

Linnea went on over the next few years to experiment with new sexual partners, to have lows and highs, and gradual and satisfying progress in her creative life. She called during several low points, depressed, self-reflective, and never suicidal. She tried antidepressant medication for a while but it "de-brained" her. She also did not want her sexual drive tampered with. She saw her old therapist occasionally. Both her children achieved independent and rewarding lives, relating to and living at times with both parents. Ultimately, she found a male partner with whom she established a long-term relationship. She never regained much weight, but her cutting stopped about two years after it began, her sense of humor blossomed, and her work, which involved creating without the use of words, became quite rewarding and fruitful.

At the end of her paper, Straker (8) discusses the cutter's lack of a secure sense of self, which one normally gains by experiencing emotions and learning, from having an attentive someone mirror and contain them, how to do so for oneself. Emotional life starts in inchoate, infantile, bodily experience. For emotions to be experienced in a human way requires interaction with other humans, repeated and sustained during human development. This is the essence of a secure attachment. Some writers refer to this as "regulation of affect." Many of our patients who have suffered from childhood abuse and neglect have not had the benefit of healthy attachment early on (11). During such an ideal emotional education, language becomes attached to emotions and is invested with some of the same representational ability. Words and their delivery become trusted vehicles of satisfying communication. A child developing with a less than secure attachment and handling neglect or abuse does not develop this facility, these tools. S/he is stuck at the level of bodily communication of feeling, which is perceived as more effective. The problem for the cutter, for all who harm themselves, and for us as their caregivers, is the lack of shared meaning. The patient is expressing an inner state, but the results of her expression are difficult for us to understand and lead us away from the patient, not toward her.

Nevertheless, many people find cutting difficult to stop. It puts boundaries and limits on turbulent feeling, as we saw from the group experience quoted above. It also does communicate something. What must our job be then? One is to see, to listen, and to try to understand. It may be helpful to recall comforting a crying infant, toddler, or young child. Another is to be a namer and a regulator. Cutting can be recognized for what it is and recognized verbally. It probably has to be given up slowly, and with a great deal of effective support. Psychotherapy, AA, support groups, inpatient psychiatric units, and obesity programs all become our partners in this endeavor. The patient needs to see the possibility of a new developmental path and to learn how to navigate it. As health care providers, we can periodically check in on how that journey is going, just as we check on medication compliance, new and healthier diets, and so on. It goes without saying that this check-in needs to be conducted in a respectful, non-judgmental fashion. Learning and change take time and effort and are probably helped by encouragement.

In medicine, we need to pay a lot of attention to the "chief complaint." This is the nugget of words (usually) which contains the essence of the problem. We should be interested, also, in what the patient does NOT say. The chief complaint may also express a great deal about the patient's self and the position they have taken regarding their problem. Linnea's chief complaint: "my therapist sent me." Perhaps she was also saying, "and here I am. I decided to come." What was she implying?

The therapist cannot ask the patient to undress and show her scars, and should not be weighing her, worrying about whether she's eating enough protein, doing alcohol levels, looking at her dental enamel, and so forth. But someone has to. In coming to see us, Linnea was agreeing to search for safety and limit-setting. Our part of the bargain is to help her create a safe space, which includes creation (and repair, when necessary) of a relationship focused on the patient's health and well-being and conducted in a positive fashion as perceived by the patient.

Often the traumatized patient's needs to do what he does far surpass his desire or ability to make healthier choices. Preventive work with all patients faces similar challenges. What makes it different with abuse survivors is the intent and intensity of the self-destruction. We all have some unhealthy inclinations and habits. But abuse survivors have a part of themselves (or incorporate a part of someone else) that is self-lethal. Someone in the past, willingly or unwillingly, lost control and invaded this person's personal/private space. Their intent was to gratify or express themselves without regard for the well-being of the victim, your patient. Your patient was assaulted. Often, to the patient, the likelihood of living through the assault was uncertain. Psychically, your patient has lived through attempted murder and has wounds to show for it. Such a patient might now regard our trying to help him recover with pity, anger, or hopelessness. Just as he was once helpless, this patient may now feel that both he and we are impotent in the face of his destructive impulses. It is important that we not succumb to that feeling. Often clinicians do, either by assuming there is nothing they can do or by assuming that this story has no relevance for the work they have been trained to do with patients. It's a "mental health problem."

In truth, however, we can say: "I am here, please don't do that, I care about you, here's what's safe and what isn't, please call if you're thinking about crossing the line." We all know patients don't have to, but we know that in asking, in setting limits, we are offering to build a positive structure with the patient and eventually, we hope, within the patient herself. How the clinician builds that space with the patient is part of his/her craft; it can be highly individual and often involves nonverbal skills. In looking back at how Linnea used our time together, I think this was perhaps the major work we did. When she had questions about how well she was doing, she checked in. When she was depressed, running out of steam, she called. The rest of it, she probably did on her own.

Perhaps I'm making this sound too simple. With each patient who harms himself, there are weighty questions. Linnea's included weight loss, the decision we had to make about how much to "work this up," the previous doctor's guess about "control" (of what?); the "cold wind of cosmic despair"; the "felt disgusting," the cuts, deep and shallow, the feeling of being not attached to earth, the implicit desire to re-attach, the bulimia and anorexia, the not eating despite appetite. We have to be alert for what danger might actually lurk for the patient. Remember, someone was/is trying to kill some part of this patient. Is the weight loss dangerous? Could there be something else wrong? Would "working up" weight loss actually be more harmful than living with it, for now? Does she think she might slice into an artery? What would that take?

We also have to accept, perhaps explicitly, that some risks lie ahead for the patient and the relationship. We don't know what will happen. Ultimately it is the patient's choice, and yet we have some responsibility. However, we have very little control. This is a moral dilemma which is not much fun.

Rosita

Rosita had been a career parochial boarding school teacher for 25 years when I first met her. She was recovering from a depression after being assigned a job at the school that was "not do-able by me." Symptoms included insomnia, low self-esteem, irritability, lots of crying. A doctor had given her amitriptyline some months prior. She was already obese and had gained 20 pounds on it. She felt "dopey" and she had just stopped it. She had somewhat controlled, long-standing hypertension and was worried about a tender lumpy area in her left breast. Both her parents had lived into old age. Coronary disease had affected some siblings, and alcohol others. She was deeply religious, single, and had never married. She denied smoking and alcohol use. She was obese, her blood pressure was in the 130/90 range, and there was a mildly worrisome area in her left breast. In the ensuing months, her breast studies were consistent with normal tissue, and she found herself presented with some extracurricular work that felt both challenging and new, and gained some measure of optimism.

Over the next few years she returned fairly regularly for physical exams, which she sometimes refused, for blood pressure follow-ups, and to report intermittent depression. At times she felt irritated with people in her living situation. She thought about retirement but needed to keep working, sometimes feeling bored. Depression returned and she took an SSRI for a while with some help, eventually stopping it after she felt better. The drug felt stigmatizing to her, and she came to feel ok without it. She reported occasional use of alcohol.

Some months later she returned for her physical exam "on edge." She had moved to a new residence within the school and was living with people who were having trouble agreeing on the basics, such as what might be served at dinner. This made her uneasy, she said. She felt her depression had lifted but was bored with her existence, again wishing to retire, again not yet able to do so. She had "an occasional drink." I saw her periodically to monitor her blood pressure.

Out of the blue one spring day, I received a hand-written note from her.

> Dear Dr. Moyer,
>
> I feel it is only right that you hear it from me, rather than (her boss), the reason why I am canceling my April appt.
>
> I was playing a game and not being honest with myself, saying I was able to cope with the situation. I began heavy drinking again on a daily basis. When I made a public ass of myself, I knew it was God's way of someone hearing my cry for help. I definitely needed it. I am an alcholic (sic). I am at (an out-of-state residential treatment center) where I will participate in a rigid, tightly scheduled program for a year. The timing is right and I am ready.
>
> When I get back, I hope I continue to have you as my Primary Care Physician.
>
> Thank you for your help.
>
> Sincerely, Rosita

When we reviewed the situation after her return, it emerged that she had been drinking, more and more heavily, for 30 years. She had never drunk alcohol until she was initiated into it by some older members of the school community, whom she now saw were alcoholic themselves. She had grown up with it, however. Her father drank regularly and beat his children with his belt when intoxicated. The incident mentioned in Rosita's letter was one of several in which she fell or was obviously intoxicated within her community. Her principal had called her to task, but by then she wanted to be "caught." "I did not want to be like my father," she said. However, for most of this time, including the times when we reviewed her alcohol history, she was in denial. She "really believed" that she was only having an occasional drink when she relayed that history to me, she said. I had believed it, too.

It eventually emerged that five years prior to her year of residential treatment, she had been on a two-week retreat and began having terrifying, repetitive dreams about a garage. She knew she didn't want to be near this garage. Then, during a massage, some memories emerged, and she had shared them with the practitioner, who was understanding. Following the retreat, she forgot, or buried everything, though dreams remained troubling.

While at the substance abuse center, which treated women only, "she discovered (again) that she had been sexually abused, got 'acquainted with her inner child,' and learned more about what the abuse had really meant to her." During treatment, she had been required to attend group sessions at which each individual had to tell their (drinking) story. She hated the group process, at one point wondering aloud, "who will be today's victim?" Using these words, one day, produced in Rosita a profound vagal response. She left the group, vomited, began shaking, encountered her counselor, and memories came rushing back. At the age of four she had been molested in a neighbor's garage by the father of a friend, a man who enticed her into the garage while her older sister stood by outside. The man promised to "play some games," then fondled and eventually raped her. When she cried, begged, and eventually vomited, he finally "got disgusted with me and told my sister to take me home and clean me up." She never told anyone; her older sister insisted that Rosita keep silent to keep the sister out of trouble, despite the girl's obvious distress and agitation. Although she grew to see how this incident had completely altered her life, she continued to have trouble participating in survivors' groups at her treatment center. Rosita often felt others' stories (often of repeated abuse) were more compelling than her own, wondering why she was there. She wanted to leave; leaders told her that her presence was important to other people, which she thought was "bull." During her year of treatment she lost 20 pounds, her blood pressure went down, and she was able to wean off all blood pressure medications. She also began to experience flashbacks and learned some ways to cope with them, though they were extremely disturbing.

Rosita has now been sober for over 20 years. Since her return, she's had times where she cannot stand to be touched and refuses some or most parts of a physical exam. She has gained back the weight she lost and has needed to return to blood pressure medication. She has flashbacks consisting of episodic, intrusive, unwanted sexual arousal, as well as intense vaginal pain. She has told me she never again will allow a colonoscopy. She has continued to live in community, for years in her original school community and now in an assisted living. She has at times felt silenced and other times spoken up courageously on matters related to mental health and addiction and been thanked for her contribution. She found the public crisis of the Catholic Church and its abusive priests very painful. Friends and relatives have died, and she has periodically been discouraged and wishing to be "taken" herself. Then she acknowledges that she is not yet ready. Still other times, she accompanies her friends in their last days and is thankful to be doing so. She attended AA for a while and periodically sees the massage therapist who knows her story and respects her boundaries. A strong relationship with God is an important part of her recovery.

Years after her initial treatment, I invited Rosita to make an educational video with me and, after consideration and with a fair amount of fear, she did it. Since then, she has regularly reminded me to make use of her sacrifice, her courage, and her contribution. "How's the book coming along?" she asks, with a little laugh. It is a potent reminder that I may not waste her precious sharing of herself and the truth she has to share with us.

Rosita's Teachings

Rosita taught me a number of lessons. One, a reminder of the well-known saw that alcoholism flourishes "under the radar." She (and I, joining her) truly believed for the first four years of our relationship that she had no problems with alcohol and that she drank only occasionally and modestly—even while she consumed ever higher quantities in private and had public episodes of drunkenness in her community. I hadn't had a clue about her inner turmoil until I got the note that April morning. Reviewing my notes, some hints were there: the feeling "on edge," the depression, the family history of drinking and violence, though that did not fully emerge until after her return. A more probing history might have raised my suspicions.

Two: alcohol, whose use grew on her, eventually became useful. It was not just experimentation and perhaps rebellion. Early on, as dreams and memories surfaced and she had trouble sleeping, it helped her cope with symptoms (insomnia, fear) that were erupting in her life.

Third: it was not wanting to be like her violent, explosive, out-of-control father that became the motivating force in her recovery. By the time she was "caught," she wanted to be caught. She entered treatment willingly. Again, we see the interweaving of violence against the self (and "turning herself in") in the service of protecting others.

Fourth, she had the luxury, due to her years of service to her school and the provision of her elders, of a full **year** to devote to the beginnings of recovery from both alcohol and an abusive childhood. Recovery will be a lifelong journey, but I am sure the gifts of time and exploration were foundational. Most people will not have the means to take a year off from earning a living, nor to pay for such services. But they will need to curtail activities and devote substantial time, energy, and money for progress to be made.

Finally, sobriety was hardly the end of her recovery, but just the beginning. Life was never easy for Rosita, either when she was drinking or when she was not. She continued to have mood swings, anger, and sometimes paralysis at injustice wherever she encountered it. But she remained a sober warrior.

Darlene

Darlene was treated in our small group practice over the course of nearly seven years. She first saw a medical resident to inquire about getting narcotics for chronic headaches. She reported a three-year history of headaches which had been worked up and felt to be "likely due to increased stress." She had just moved to our area from out of state. She was using one or two Percocet every four hours when she had a headache; these might occur daily, or not at all for weeks. She had tried beta blockers as prevention with no help. She had been at the ER the week prior to her visit with the resident. Darlene noted that this was a "stressful and unrewarding experience" and wanted a doctor at our practice so that would not have to happen again. The resident did not document whether or not he had checked the ER note. He raised the question of drug-seeking behavior but "truly" doubted it. A neurologic exam was normal. The resident noted that "she has tried everything in the past and that has not helped." What exactly he meant by that is not clear.

Darlene saw a covering physician and sought and received 30 Percocets; then, three months later, she had a first appointment with the internist to whom she was now assigned. She complained of exhaustion, dizziness, trouble concentrating, and "persistent headaches, which are relieved with over-the-counter medications." She had been smoking since the age of 13. She was encouraged to contemplate stopping this. She stated she had had a nonprofit job for the past six years (though she had only moved here less than a year ago).

The two got together a month later for a complete exam. Headaches, the failure of prior meds, the possibility of Imitrex, and depression were discussed. Her fatigue was gone. She lived alone. She didn't want to quit smoking. She was a sports fan. Her mother had died of cancer, and a maternal uncle of suicide. She was the youngest of three. Her general and neurologic exams were normal save for obesity; she was described as "jolly and talkative" and was given a trial of Imitrex and 45 Percocets "with one refill" along with a request to follow up in six months.

Darlene was seen eight times over the next 10 months, five of them for pain syndromes (mostly, though not all, headache) and got four Percocet prescriptions. There was a growing concern about the headaches and narcotic use, and she had a neurology referral midway through the year. She told the neurologist she'd been born in a different state than she told us. She was given advice about lifestyle modification and a small number of benzodiazepines. She did not find any of this helpful and later in the year was given a referral to another neurologist at a local holistic practice, to whom she never went.

The following year, she rather abruptly had a new issue. She complained of several months of neck and arm pain and was felt to have cervical nerve root impingement. An MRI showed mild to moderate cervical spine degenerative disease. Darlene was referred to neurosurgery, after requesting and getting thirty more Percocets. The neurosurgeon did not send any notes, but her workup revealed carpal tunnel syndrome, for which she got more narcotics, and treatment.

Migraines returned within two months. Her primary care physician met with her at her behest to discuss a "situation" between her and her boss which had "escalated." In the next four months, she got 60 more Percocets from our office. Sinus x-rays were negative. Her doctor planned a longer time to revisit the headaches and look again at non-narcotic treatment, but when Darlene returned, she said she'd gotten her boss fired, was herself promoted, and "is very happy about it." An informal assessment and contract for 10 Percocets per month was established.

The contract was strengthened verbally several months later (same amount) at a time when the patient was doing well and had planned with her primary care physician to taper off of her SSRI. In fact, however, the contract was violated by both patient and clinic staff; she seems to have gotten more than twice that amount during this year. Meanwhile, pain in her right hand inexplicably returned; she saw a hand surgeon who could not explain her symptoms anatomically, was concerned about narcotic use, and referred her to a pain clinic. She saw a neurosurgeon who, after repeat imaging, did not feel her neck anatomy had anything to do with the pain and referred her back to hand and pain providers. She was apparently begun on some sort of neck injections, though no notes from the pain clinic ever arrived at our office.

The following year, Darlene seemed more in crisis. There was a phone call after the holidays stating she was using "10 to 15" Percocets **per day,** worrying about liver damage. She lost her job a month later and was unemployed for months, reporting some financial help from her father and continuing to request Percocets at intervals, now for unclear indications. Midway through the year, she saw her primary doctor and resumed treatment with the SSRI. Later in the year she had subjective left arm weakness without objective findings, was seen again by neurosurgery—who, after exam, stated that "the fluctuation of her pain syndrome argues against a fixed anatomic abnormality . . . I would not consider any surgical approach for pain management" and discharged her from care. By the end of the year, she seemed to be getting about 30 Percocets per month and described herself as "living with chronic pain."

In the fifth year with our practice, Darlene's primary care doctor moved for family reasons and relocated her practice about 40 miles away. I and a physician assistant took over Darlene's primary care. She called once looking for extra Percocet, and after I refused, then called monthly as originally agreed upon. Later that winter, at our first visit together, she described "chronic thoracic pain" that rendered her "unable to sit up" without a Percocet. It had been going on for four years and began after a whiplash injury, she stated. "I'm a chronic pain patient," she said. None of this had previously been documented in the chart. At the end of the interview, she asked for Percocet. She was nine days early, and I told her I would not give them to her. I had decided not to explore the requests for additional drugs, the varied stories about pain, or anything else, yet.

There followed several visits with the physician assistant, which now focused back on neck pain, on requests for earlier and higher doses of the narcotic, and which resulted in a repeat cervical MRI showing no nerve or nerve root impingement. Neurologic exam showed no deficits. Darlene refused to retry physical therapy or any new meds or modalities. She continued to test the limits of her contract, eventually giving up on the PA, whose limit-setting made her feel "treated quite poorly." She told me she suffered "bouts of debilitating pain, relieved by pain medication" due to "cervical disc disease . . . as indicated on the 3 MRIs." She complained of being made to feel "like a defendant in a murder trial . . . and questions were put to me so as to make me feel as though I was being deceptive in my responses, perhaps trying to get her to furnish me with prescription drugs unnecessarily."

At this point, the PA and I were concerned about not furthering what appeared to be substance misuse or abuse. I hoped to begin some more explicit discussion; but Darlene needed eye surgery, had a preop visit, then shortly thereafter had to go to the ER for an acute appendicitis. Surgery revealed a micro-perforation: her course was either rapid, or her own recognition was delayed. There was one note from her surgeon in the post-op period refusing her request for additional pain meds for post-op pain. She did seem to be recovering normally by the time I saw her, and I gave her her monthly refill (for a syndrome I still did not understand). She called for the next six months for Percocet on a regular basis, on one occasion calling four days early and being denied until the proper date, without a complaint.

The following spring, she finally came to me for her first long examination. Her childhood was turbulent. Her parents separated when she was six and then divorced. Her mother remarried. Her uncle suicided in her teen years. Later in her adolescence, the patient, her mother, and stepfather moved to a new state, following her stepfather's job. "Her stepfather became sexually forward with her in her teen years," I wrote. Her mother contracted cancer when the patient was 21 and still living at home. "When I wouldn't 'put out' as a young woman when my mother was dying, he (the stepfather) pitched me out of the house," Darlene reported. Her biologic father paid her living expenses for a while, and she got some employment training. Her mother died when Darlene was 26, and she then moved to a different state and worked for a decade or so. She had moved to our area to be closer to an old friend, and that is when we had met her. She was currently working in a local nonprofit and lived alone.

Exam showed acne scars, obesity, and the recent appendectomy scar. She was "talkative and engaging." She told me that smoking was her "only vice and addiction." That was my opening. We discussed the Percocet use and its increase over the years for both headache and unexplained neck pain. She liked Percocet because it "relieved the pain" and had "no side effects." We agreed for her to increase her dose of amitriptyline. Screening labs were ordered, and we made no change in the Percocet dose.

Four months later, she came in because she was "getting worse." She was taking amitriptyline rather randomly. She had bouts of increased pain several times per week in her neck and arms. The pain bore no relation to activity or position. The pain caused her to leave work, or to be ineffective or make mistakes, she said, and she worried about losing her job. She wanted an extra narcotic prescription. On exam, she had findings consistent with myofascial pain, and a negative neurological exam. I suggested various non-narcotics we could try, and some further physical therapy. We then discussed the dangers of substance misuse, and addiction. She was "quite surprised that Percocet could cause drug addiction . . . in fact, when I take Percocet, I get no high at all." I told her that (addiction) was probably the worst possible outcome of all of this, but I hoped that it never happened, and that my hope was to get her off all narcotics. She was given a physical therapy referral, no additional Percocet, and told to follow up in one month.

The next day she called, stating she was going to return to her previous doctor—the one from our clinic who had moved 40 miles away. She called two weeks later, giving verbal permission for her records to be sent to that office. A day later, that doctor's office called, saying Darlene was there and asking for records. We requested written permission before sending anything. A call a few weeks later to my former colleague revealed that she had not actually seen her.

Several days later, my front office received a call from a friend of the patient's, stating that Darlene was found dead in her apartment. Her case went to the Medical Examiner. The death certificate reads "cardiac arrest" due to "atherosclerotic coronary artery disease." She was 46 years old. I requested her autopsy report from the state. I never received it.

Substance Misuse and Abuse

Darlene's case, laid out in narrative detail above, may feel familiar. It took so long to grasp what might be happening. She presented contradictory details. Multiple providers were involved. Many were made uneasy by her behavior. Her reports had many loose ends. We never knew what the truth might be. And we are left with a terrible ending, with the truth not necessarily provided even with the autopsy. The headaches and intermittent neck pain certainly did not suggest coronary disease. Her 33 years of smoking were certainly relevant here. But could this have actually been an overdose death or, like her uncle, a suicide?

I present Darlene's course, feeling in good measure uncertainties and worries, to help us consider some of the ramifications of substance abuse, its connection to childhood abuse and neglect, and its treatment. Certainly, one cause has to be a tremendous increase in narcotic prescribing by US providers over recent decades (decreasing now due to public and governmental pressures, and professional self-discipline (12). For instance, between 1997 and 2007, retail sales of oxycodone (in grams) went from roughly 4.5 million, to almost 43 million. More than 80% of the world's global production of oxycodone is consumed in the United States. These drugs are easily available in our country, and abundantly so. In 2009, about 40% of opioid prescriptions were written by providers in general practice and internal medicine, far more than the numbers written by pain clinic providers, physiatrists, dentists, or orthopedists. Unintentional overdose deaths from opioids began surpassing those from cocaine or heroin in 2001. Since then, the gap has widened. The addition of fentanyl to the illegal drug supply, and the psychosocial effects of the Covid-19 pandemic, have deepened our country's troubles with opioid addiction.

Building an evidence base for universal screening of primary care patients for substance use disorders has been difficult (13). Instead, providers encounter a scenario similar to Darlene's, in which the question repeatedly surfaces and disappears, based on the patient's behavior, lifestyle, or use of medication. Bonhomme et al. (14) write of some of these warning signs, including repeated running out of medications, doctor shopping, claims of lost prescriptions, possession of multiple opioid prescription bottles, or theft of prescription pads. He also warns of mood and personality changes, drug side effects, and concerning behaviors around medications, including taking more drugs than prescribed. Finally. social changes including poor job or school performance, changes in friend networks, or absenteeism may be signs of a progressive substance abuse problem.

Shapiro et al. (13) write helpfully for those in primary care, differentiating hazardous use (e.g., driving or decision-making with drugs in the system) from substance abuse, and that from substance dependence. Substance abuse is defined as a "maladaptive pattern of substance use leading to clinically significant impairment or distress" within a given year involving at least one of the following:

not fulfilling work/home/school obligations
repeated "hazardous" use (e.g. driving under the influence)
recurrent legal issues involving substance
continued use despite social issues caused by using substance (e.g., spousal objection)

Substance dependence he also defines as a "maladaptive pattern" over a year but with at least three of seven accompanying features: tolerance; withdrawal; taking progressively larger amounts; unsuccessful efforts to cut down; expenditure of a lot of time and effort in getting, using, and recovering from use of the substance; withdrawal from other social activities to spend more time with the substance; or continued use despite knowledge of its negative health effects.

I was unaware of these distinctions during our care of Darlene. What made me and other caregivers uneasy were the blithe use of narcotics for conditions for which the majority of the populace does not use them; the repeated requests for early or extra refills; the "jolly" mien contrasting with the desperate; the job instability and crises. In retrospect, Darlene also had an amazing ability to have life events occur just as confrontation was planned, so that her narcotic use marched along for months or years without conscious consideration between doctor and patient.

Truth was flimsy, or filmy, between us. Was Darlene sexually abused as a teen and young adult? Here I think we have to take her story, which was composed of multiple traumas—early divorce between parents (why and involving what?), moving, family suicide, relative isolation among siblings, maternal illness and death, and the stepfather's advances toward her—at face value. We cannot know more until she tells us, and what she tells us gives us a picture of disruption and loss during her formative years. Much of the story emerged late in her care. A thorough social history taken earlier in her care, including developmental events, would have been a useful "red flag."

Teicher and Samson (15) have recently proposed "that affected individuals with childhood maltreatment constitute a critically distinct subtype across depressive, anxiety and substance use disorders. . . . the maltreated subtype may be thought of as a phenotypic specialization (phenocopy) resulting from environmental experience. . . . Why focus on maltreatment? Because it is maltreatment rather than exposure to other stressors, such as natural disasters, that consistently presents as the antecedent to psychopathology." Reviewing studies of individuals with major depression, anxiety disorders, and substance use, they show a consistently higher incidence of all three among patients with history of childhood maltreatment. Importantly, the depressions that emerge in maltreated subjects appear to be qualitatively different than individuals without maltreatment. They are more treatment-resistant, they may not respond well to drugs, and they may respond better to cognitive behavioral therapy than individuals without maltreatment. They cite neurobiological underpinnings of these differences, mainly the reduction in hippocampal volume among patients with histories of childhood maltreatment, arguing that these phenomenological and anatomical differences constitute evidence for a distinct "ecophenotype."

Childhood maltreatment at least triples the risk for drug dependence, though many confounding factors complicate the relationship. As in the case with depression, the illness does not look the same. The actual illness may begin earlier in life and be associated with increased tendencies for risky sexual behaviors, incarceration, greater subjective distress, and more personality disorders. Neuroimaging research has suggested that maltreated substance abusers show deficits of dopamine systems and deficiencies in operation of the orbitofrontal cortex and anterior cingulate gyrus, which "may underlie the patterns of compulsive and impulsive behaviors that characterize addiction." Whether these changes are seen in the majority of maltreated individuals (i.e., both with and without substance abuse) has yet to be seen, but the anatomic basis for risk may be seen here.

Teicher and Samson review a variety of structural/functional differences in the brains of people with histories of childhood maltreatment, and also review the findings that different parts of the brain are susceptible to disarray due to abuse at different times during childhood development. They also note that there may be delayed effects, with alterations that we might label as disease, not showing up for years after the anatomic changes have been wrought. They point out the need for different and better treatments for this subtype, noting that "integrative trauma-focused treatments . . . for maltreated individuals with substance abuse . . . are more helpful than standard treatments, though results are far from ideal."

Unclear also was the extent of Darlene's use and accumulation of opioids (or other substances). During the time of her care, our state did not have a prescription monitoring program, although we do now. Use of such a program could theoretically have alerted her caregivers to her issues if she was receiving prescriptions from multiple providers. We didn't know what we did not know. Variable data exist, however, on the effect of such programs in preventing opioid mortality, with some studies showing a slowing of the rise of deaths and others, not. Gordon et al. (16) reviews some recent encouraging studies using buprenorphine-naloxone in patients with substance use disorders and chronic pain, demonstrating "favorable addiction and pain outcomes" among such patients, in contrast to worries of some that pain will not be adequately controlled in such patients. Gordon et al. also uncovered data showing that integration of addiction care into high quality (as perceived by the patient) primary care treatment is associated with lower substance use severity. This and other studies would argue for the integration into primary care of substance abuse treatment with other chronic illnesses, but presupposes adequate staffing and expertise (psychiatry, social work, security) to help the primary providers. These are elements that exist in the conception of a patient-centered medical home, though many if not most current practices lack such staffing. In addition, mechanisms to pay for such staffing are sorely lacking.

Best and Lubman (17) recently reviewed literature on recovery from substance abuse, a goal which may seem ephemeral to clinicians on the front lines. They argue for long-term (years) treatment, conceptualizing drug abuse as an illness like diabetes or hypertension with a years-long if not lifelong time span. They present evidence that "58% of addicted individuals will eventually achieve lasting recovery," defined in several ways. These include the notions of a lifestyle voluntarily chosen, involving sobriety and control over substance use and interconnected with personal health and participation in social welfare of self and others. They note the critical importance of "other people" in recovery programs, especially "abstinence specific social support"—which must complement what medical treatment can do. They note that full recovery may take over a quarter of a century and note implications for those of us in general practice. They emphasize the importance of safety, a place to live, freedom from undue physical distress, and good quality information about what routes towards sobriety are available. These are the precursors. But during the actual treatment, we must "instill hope that the individual can recover and be mindful that their relationship (with us) can be a critical 'turning point' in the patient's recovery journey; act as a 'bridge' to groups and individuals who successfully model recovery; and involve family members in supporting their recovery journey."

We never even got started on any of this with Darlene.

Reflections on Recovery

Linnea, Rosita, and Darlene each have their individual stories, but with many features in common. They all highlight the crucial importance of safety in the doctor–patient alliance. They highlight the different meanings of "safety" to doctor and patient and how the mutual conception changes through time, as relationship, truth, and healing evolve or do not. They highlight the sense in which woven in with the harmful behavior is a self-structure experienced and believed by the patient as real, very hard to give up, and quite protective. Yet this is a self-structure that ultimately is based on a lie, which is woven in with the abandonment of memories and experiences. They highlight our relative impotence to help our trauma patients without what AA might term our "higher powers"—the courage of the patient to trust, the will of both doctor and patient to bear the truth and to know what needs to be known, and the strength and enough wisdom to do these things together.

What can we say about safety? Judith Herman (18) states that it is integral to the first stage of a therapeutic recovery from trauma of any sort, and stresses the importance of naming the problem, establishing the locus of control in the client, and working with her to create a safe environment for herself. Linnea and Rosita had options for a safe space, and treatment, and Linnea went on to change her own personal environment substantially. Darlene may perhaps have fled from the beginning of basic knowledge; I believe that safety was never hers.

These women's stories show us that to deal with abuse is to deal with the possibility and reality of death. Although our living patients have survived physically, there is a part of them that knows death, that would rather be dead than face the truth; that could cooperate with death, and that this part is much nearer than we would like to know.

None of these patients had integrated whatever knowledge they had of their past sexual trauma when I first met them. The self-harm in which they were engaged was testimony to that. But even knowing that they were hurting themselves, much less what it was related to, was sometimes difficult to unravel. Linnea was cutting herself and losing weight. She was sent (I believe—though the therapist never called me) to "rule out organic causes" and perhaps to establish a safe floor for her weight. In addition, there was the strong family history of cancer. Was she ill with a malignancy? Rosita's drinking flourished for years—decades—without her naming it within herself or being able to truthfully answer a question about her drinking. She also elicited no concern in me or other providers about this as a possibility. Darlene, as has been illustrated, created clouds of suspicion and confusion in most providers about her drug use. However, she had the ability to slip through everyone's fingers. Her diagnoses and pains changed, and her use flourished as these were "treated" and chased after. Once confronted, she professed complete surprise about the addictive nature of opiates. Was she being manipulative and untruthful? Or was she living within a lie that she felt she could not live without?

In all cases, I believe, these patients would have been safer had I, along with all their other doctors and caregivers, had greater familiarity with and suspicion of the workings of violence in our society. In day-to-day terms, that might be as easy (and difficult) as taking a trauma history, along with a family and social history, as soon as practical. There can be direct questions about situations past and present of fear, harm, neglect, and assault. There can be notations of how the patient conducts his answers (dissociative behavior, evasiveness, contradictions). And there can and should be direct knowledge by the provider of the public health information given to us to use by Fellitti et al.—the knowledge that the more adverse childhood experiences an individual has had, the worse their health is likely to be. We can practice knowing that violence is rife and that self-harm, too, is rife, and that our indices of suspicion must be high for both.

In self-harm, the patient is (re-)traumatizing herself. She is the only one who can stop it. Knowing it is happening, acknowledgment in a relationship, is the beginning, but it must be clear to the patient that stopping it is her job, not ours. Much as we might want to, we cannot rescue such people and will in fact hurt them and us in trying. What then is our job? After identification, there is standard bearing, help with reliable resources, a firm bottom line, and the building or rebuilding of a trusting, respectful, compassionate relationship that incorporates our new knowledge of the patient. Alcoholism goes on the problem list. At each encounter we don't neglect to ask, encourage, and redirect, as appropriate. It is our job to search out and maintain a wide variety of community resources—addiction programs, battered women's shelters, self-help groups, trauma-informed therapists, inpatient units, eating programs, and the like, to which we can refer patients when they are ready. Recovery from trauma involves sudden swings in mood and self-resolve; we must establish with patients what we will do if they cannot keep themselves safe, and define what that means in their particular case. Day-to-day encouragement, sometimes feeling like verbal droning to us, matters much more than we know.

The primary care provider has the difficult task of observing the patient's self-proscribed limits while advising them on their health. People with abuse histories who are recovering will often develop some clear ideas about what can or cannot be done to them. (Before recovery, such people may just dissociate and allow the thing to be done, or have a catastrophic, shocking response, e.g., during a colonoscopy.) On the one hand, it is imperative that these wishes be respected. Linnea wanted her sister out of the consulting room. Rosita refused exams on multiple occasions, or "nothing below the waist." These limits can be observed, and doing that can help the patient feel safe and respected. On the other hand, some limits must at least be probed. Rosita refused to repeat her colonoscopy at the time she was due, saying "she's convinced she would not undertake any cancer treatment if cancer were found, including simple surgery." "I pray to be taken." There may be a part of every survivor that would rather die than face humiliation, or re-traumatization—however it is defined. That part can be reached. Reaching such a part is the work of an ally, which is what a provider becomes. We must always be judging how hard and how far to push or probe.

But perhaps most important, in a long-term primary care relationship, one must incorporate the new knowledge of the patient in a way that validates who they now are. In showing us their scars, in saying "I binge" instead of "but doctor, I hardly eat at all," patients are a step closer to a truth about all of their existence, including what befell them in the past. Taking this step, when trauma has been involved, brings up powerful feelings of shame, fear, rage, and helplessness, even when the trauma is not remembered or linked. It takes great courage on the part of people. Normalizing the feelings and acknowledging their courage and strength at facing them, walking that walk with them—all of this matters.

We never knew who Darlene really was. I never knew who Rosita was either, until she came to terms with her addiction. When I asked her, years later, how it could have been that for four years, during which she had told me she did not drink much, that was the truth that lived between us, she said "I really did not think that I did. I felt that I **was** that person I described to you."

References

1. "Torture," from MIRACLE FAIR by Wislawa Szymborska, translated by Joanna Trzeciak, p. 46. Copyright © 2001 by Joanna Trzeciak. Used by permission of W.W. Norton & Company, Inc., 2002.
2. Vailliant G, *The Natural History of Alcoholism*, Harvard University Press, 1983.
3. Reece J, "Female survivors of abuse attending A & E with self-injury," *Accident and Emergency Nursing* 6(3): 133–138, 1998.
4. Felitti VJ, "Adverse childhood experiences and adult health," *Academic Pediatrics* 9(3): 131–132, 2009.
5. Starecheski L, "Ten Questions Some Doctors Are Afraid to Ask," Podcast on NPR, March 3, 2015.
6. Ibid., March 3, 2015.
7. Felitti VJ and Anda RF, "The relationship of adverse childhood experiences to adult medical disease, psychiatric disorders and sexual behavior: implications for healthcare," in Lanius R, Vermetten E, and Pain C, (eds.), *The Hidden Epidemic: The Impact of Early Life Trauma on Health and Disease*, pp. 77–87. Cambridge University Press, 2011.
8. Straker G, "Signing with a scar: understanding self-harm," *Psychoanalytic Dialogues*, 16(1): 93–112, 2006.
9. Ford JD, Fallot, RD, and Harris M, "Group Therapy," in Courtois CA and Ford, JD, (eds.), *Treating Complex Traumatic Stress Disorders*, pp. 415–440. Guilford Press, 2009.
10. Teicher M, Rabi K, Sheu Y, Seraphin S, Andersen S, Anderson C, et al., "Neurobiology of Childhood Trauma and Adversity," in Lanius and Vermetten, *The Hidden Epidemic*, 2009.
11. Brown D, "Assessment of Attachment and Abuse History, and Adult Attachment Style," in Courtois and Ford, *Treating Complex Distress Orders*, 2009.
12. Manchikanti L, Helm II S, Fellows B, Janata J, Pampati V, Grider J, and Boswell M, "Opioid epidemic in the United States," *Pain Physician* 15(3 Suppl): ES9–ES3, 2012.
13. Shapiro B, Coffa D, and McCance-Katz E, "A primary care approach to substance misuse," *American Family Physician* 88(2): 113–121, 2013.
14. Bonhomme J, Shim R, Gooden R, Tyus, D, and Rust G, "Opioid addiction and abuse in primary care practice: a comparison of methadone and buprenorphine as treatment options," *Journal of the National Medical Association* 104(0): 342–350, 2012.

15. Teicher M and Samson J, "Childhood maltreatment and psychopathology: A case for ecophenotypic variants and clinically and neurobiologically distinct subtypes," *American Journal of Psychiatry*, 170(10): 1114–1133, October, 2013.
16. Gordon A, Bertholet N, McNeely J, Starrels J, Tetrault J, Walley A, "Update in addiction medicine for the generalist," *Addiction Science & Clinical Practice* 8:18, 2013.
17. Best D and Lubman D, "The recovery paradigm, A model of hope and change for alcohol and drug addiction," *Australian Family Physician* 41(8) 593–597, 2012.
18. Herman J, *Trauma and Recovery*, Chapter 8, BasicBooks, HarperCollins, 1992.

7
Trauma and the Body

> *"Why were you asking him about all of that stuff?"*
>
> *—a second-year medical student*

> *"The patient is stable and the cause, while unknown, seems to be of no significant concern."*
>
> *—a second-year medical student write-up of the same case*

Introduction

I assisted for years in teaching a course for medical students whose purpose was to impart the skills of interviewing and examining patients. Students early in their 7 to10 years of medical training are exposed in depth to ill patients and learn to take a history and perform a physical examination. One fall some time ago, we began the course anew. I was mentoring two young men, and our patient was Mr. D, an 88-year-old former truck driver who had entered the hospital because of the new onset of intractable vomiting.

The students together found out that Mr. D, several weeks prior, had begun vomiting significant portions of every meal, without pain, fever, weight loss, change in meds, or other symptoms. One of his children had prevailed upon him to seek medical attention after his symptoms had failed to improve spontaneously. The vomiting had stopped immediately upon hospitalization, with no specific therapeutic intervention, five days prior, and he was now eating solid food without any trouble. The students were unsure what tests or therapy had been administered and knew little about differential diagnosis at this point in their education. They did find out that he was a wounded veteran, that he complained about a lot of anxiety, that he had been married and had a couple of children, and that many years ago he had suffered a severe crush injury requiring months of rehabilitation but from which he eventually returned to work and normal well-being. They were impressed with his having shrapnel still embedded in his neck, which the patient said limited his neck motions, and the fact that he was an avid sports fan. They described him as "mentally alert." He had never had this vomiting problem before.

We returned to the bedside to find out more about Mr. D's life. He was a muscular man who appeared younger than his stated age. He did not look at us while giving history, instead staring into the immediate distance while answering our questions with a bit of ironic distance as well. He could not explain his stance (I asked), though the students thought it might have been the shrapnel that made him do this. He clearly enjoyed the interchange, the students' youth, and the bits of humor involved in being a trainer for ones just starting out in their craft. He kept a straight face while doing so. His dry replies frequently made the students laugh. He **was** "mentally alert."

We all sat down next to Mr. D. After fishing around for a while, I asked him more about what was going on before this started. Two weeks before he began vomiting, the son of a neighbor, to whom he was very close, died suddenly. Mr. D had been "like a father" to the deceased. The wife of the deceased had come to the house to tell the patient of the death, and it was an enormous, sad shock. Over the coming days, the wife had developed a plan to bury her husband's body in the family gravesite which *the patient* had already purchased. He strongly objected to this plan, telling her, "That's MY site!" (At this point in the story, the older man in the next bed guffawed with understanding.) As things developed, she then had her husband cremated, took the ashes, dug a hole without permission on the patient's burial ground, and put them in. When he had heard about this, he told us, he had rolled his eyes, thought the 88-year-old equivalent of "whatever"... shaken his head... and a few days later had begun vomiting.

My two students and I examined Mr. D's mouth and abdomen (learning most of the physical exam was still ahead of the students). We found nothing remarkable. We thanked him for his time and instruction of us. He invited us back "any time" and told another little joke, and we left.

The students were uncomfortable, mystified, and confused, and well they should have been. What place did this history have in this illness? Why would I suggest that the stories were related? What about the tests which had been done (which we had not accessed) and what they showed? What role did this history have in Mr. D's diagnosis, treatment, and recovery?

As I re-read this incident, I also wonder: what role did this story have in the education of these two medical students? Given the quote from one of their write-ups, above, I suspect it became a buried byproduct, an incomprehensible, non-digested bit of information relegated to the dusty attics of memory. The students had had a year of intensive instruction in human gross and cellular anatomy, physiology, and pathophysiology, imparted in Cartesian fashion. What basis did they have for understanding or even inquiring into this person's body and mind relationships? Speaking for myself, I don't have a theoretical understanding of the physical relationship between his taking in of this beloved younger man's death (experience of shock, grief), the man's wife's feeling that her husband needed to lie in death near our patient's family, our patient's strong objections to her plans ("that's my place!!"), his reaction to her solution, and his subsequent vomiting. All I have is his story, a feeling that all is related, and the supposition that were I this man's doctor rather than a doctor-educator meeting him for one time, I would have woven this story, this reaction, into the basis of our subsequent relationship—unless another, better explanation ensued. I doubt it would have.

The medical student's history and the patient's behavior gave us a picture of a resilient human being. He was 88 years old. He had survived injury during war. He had miraculously survived a major injury in his work. He displayed advanced adaptive defenses of humor, irony, and altruism. While he did not "meet" us openly, this was perhaps healthy, given the students' novice status. What happens to individuals and their bodies when they are not as well constructed, when something or someone in their life comes to crush them, and succeeds?

The "Speech" of the Body, and Treatment

The body, and complaints about the body, are the "currency" of internal medicine. A foundation of our practice is that disease and disorder give rise to changes, which are experienced and expressed as symptoms and signs, and communicated to health care providers who can recognize and sort such symptoms physiologically into diseases. We then reach into various toolboxes to try remedies and stay in contact with patients to see how those remedies are working. It is comforting to have a chapter in a textbook to refer to, a physiology to explain what we are dealing with.

Many of the patients that generalists see in the clinic and hospital complain of bodily symptoms we cannot sort through in such a neat fashion. Ten symptoms—abdominal pain, back pain, chest pain, dizziness, fatigue, headache, insomnia, numbness, shortness of breath, and swelling –account for up to 40% of primary care visits, but generalists can only find a biological explanation for about one-fourth of them (1). In practicing primary care, we are working at the limits of our understanding of the effects of inflammation, injury, infection, vascular disease, neoplasm, and emotional trauma on the tissues of the body and the nervous system. Exciting research is ongoing at the molecular and brain–body level, but practically, we are left to our own devices to find a way to work with people's day-to-day problems.

About half of patients with inexplicable somatic symptoms have experienced significant childhood trauma (2). Others have had other experiences, but they may have in common the unexamined story, the untold history hiding in the body.

"Medically unexplained symptoms" (MUS) have become the subject of research. Some studies deal with how doctors and patients think about such symptoms, how they react to their presence, how they both learn (or not) to cope with them. Somatization, another term for the experience of the client facing non-understood disease-associated symptoms, has been defined by Singh (3) as "the tendency to experience, conceptualize and communicate mental states and distress as physical symptoms and altered body states." Singh thus advances the proposition that a medically unexplained symptom might be one or several feelings or memories in disguise. Stone and Clarke (4) emphasizes that somatizers do not choose their symptoms consciously (in contrast to malingerers). Rather, they experience an array of physical symptoms and are compelled due to their severity to bring them to a medical encounter. Somatizers are uncomfortable, worried, frightened people. Somatizers may experience a bodily feeling where another person might have an emotional reaction. Sometimes, the chosen symptom has personal meaning or cultural significance (4). Patients do not define themselves as somatizers—doctors do.

There is a danger, of which primary caregivers are well aware, in lumping all symptoms we don't understand into this one basket and labeling all patients who have them as somatizers. With some years of practice, all clinicians will have the repeated experience of the odd symptom being the herald of an organic disease. In addition, there are lots of rare diseases with peculiar manifestations.

On the other hand, there will be a great and frequent loss of medical effectiveness if the provider does not understand in his heart and soul something about the origins of what we call medically unexplained symptoms. In addition, I don't think these symptoms are so far out of the ken of what we do every day with people with organic processes. The key lies in understanding the difference between the disease and the illness. The disease concept encompasses our understanding of the physiologic or biochemical basis of a malady. The illness, however, represents the sum of all the disturbance and suffering in a patient's life caused by the malady. As Eric Cassell (5) has pointed out, suffering caused by disease is individual and highly personal. Not just pain and disability, but interpersonal disturbance, self-concept, and moral and spiritual dimensions are involved. Tending to and understanding these aspects of all human distress is one of the cores of primary care work, and one basis of its challenges and rewards.

The twentieth century saw an explosion of physiologic and biochemical knowledge about the body, and medical training underwent a parallel revolution after the Flexner report of 1910. By mid-century, the federal government was on board with the creation of the National Institute of Health, and the funding of residency training. Science now rules, and from what we hear about the past, we should and do welcome it. Unfortunately, this primacy has had the effect of minimizing and sullying the reputation of the parallel work of intuition, linguistics, body language, and the exploration of stories. Thus, the phrase "medically unexplained symptom" takes on a certain pejorative sense, perhaps reflecting the difficulty many clinicians, generalists and specialists alike, have in listening to such symptoms. The difficulty is multifactorial, as we shall see. The somatizer often finds herself belittled, second-class, unwelcome. She has the symptoms that cause specialists to suggest that a patient "should see your primary care doctor about that"—often with relief.

A clarification is in order here. Clinicians see many people every day with unexplained symptoms. Many of these are short-lived. They go away with time or reassurance, or they become part of the fabric of aging or chronic disease. When we speak of people with medically unexplained symptoms, we are talking of those who return repeatedly with unchanging or slowly evolving complaints for which no organic explanation can be found after thorough evaluation. Studies indicate that such symptoms seen in a primary care setting may last longer than those caused by organic disease; and that people with unexplained symptoms have as poor health ratings as those who have organic disease (6).

The phrase "medically unexplained symptoms" says as much, however, about medical science as it does about "somatization." Our science is woefully deficient at understanding and explaining entire realms of human experience. Nevertheless, we have to define a useful path forward for patients and clinicians alike. In general medicine, this means developing a wide-ranging understanding of the patient, recognizing patterns, conveying whatever truths we have found to the patient, and developing a plan. The plan may provide relief. But what most importantly provides relief, according to Peters et al. (7), is the sense that the doctor can be trusted to try to understand and to be thorough. Working on this type of partnership is *what we need to do*, whether or not science has provided us with tools for understanding what may be going on. Furthermore, it is in the context of this type of relationship that a patient is more likely to offer emotional cues and to share some of their already developed psychological understanding with their provider. The alert physician, in a relationship of earned trust, may attend to such cues, decreasing the likelihood of a "somatic outcome."

This work is much harder to do when the patient's communication is non-linear or cryptic, which is often the case. When tests show "nothing wrong"— or worse, red herrings—we can be waylaid by the patient's disappointment or our need to provide further follow-up and investigation. This is one reason why general practice is among the most difficult specialties a clinician can choose. Doing it well involves using all of our personal powers—intellectual, organizational, emotional, physical, and spiritual.

A variety of studies carried out in doctor–patient situations involving medically unexplained symptoms explores doctors' strategies and behavior in these murky waters. Epstein et al. (8) studied physicians' responses to two standardized patients in Rochester, NY: one patient had a typical esophageal reflux (GERD) story; the other presented "concerns that physicians would not easily be able to fit into a clear unifying diagnostic category". Using the Measure of Patient-Centered Communication, they catalogued physician responses. They found that doctors were less likely to explore and validate symptoms with the MUS patients, and that they spent no more time or effort exploring the psychosocial issues with the MUS patient than they did with the GERD patient. They speculated that ignorance, a sense of lack of time, and attitude may have underpinned this behavior. (One can ask, is GERD, or any other illness, a true control, in that much of its symptomatology is governed by patient behaviors and reactions which have their root in the stresses of daily life and in the patient's habitual response to them.)

Olde Hartman et al. used focus groups of 22 general practitioners (GPs) to explore their knowledge and perceptions about patients with medically unexplained symptoms, and about their relationships with these patients (9). These doctors felt that explanations of symptoms were important but related that they had trouble actually explaining to the patient what was going on. They seemed to lack a model, although the author pointed out that such models exist. According to these practitioners, they evolved several types of relationships over time, characterized as mutual alliance, ambivalent alliance, and non-alliance. In the first, the doctor realized "at a certain moment in your approach of the patient, when a patient has had all diagnostic procedures and many referrals, then comes the moment when one realizes: this is the only way this patient can live. Consequently, I let him consult me sporadically, even without complaints." In the second, the general practitioners went along with similar ritualistic behavior but felt disgruntled by it, stating for instance "that in these situations the patient is in control of the situation." Finally, a few indicated no alliance with the patient when these symptoms dominated. One doctor stated: "The patient is the one with the problem, it is not my problem, it is your problem, and you have to solve that with the social worker." The vast majority, however, seemed to feel that it was their responsibility to build and maintain a relationship with the patient, with the symptoms as a nexus.

Salmon et al. (10) studied hundreds of audiotaped recordings of consultations of patients' presentations of medically unexplained symptoms to their doctors, looking for which factors influenced a "somatic intervention"—drugs, tests, referrals. Providers' experiences of such encounters might predict that it was pressure from patients which led to medical intervention. Salmon found instead that "extended symptom presentation"—the patient elaborating on symptoms or adding more symptoms— was predictive of the provider taking such action. Longer consultations were also associated with more somatic interventions. (Whether appointment length was due to a doctor's interests, involvement with the patient, skills, efficiency, or patient complexity was not addressed in this study). Interestingly, patients' psychosocial talk, either in relation to their symptoms, *or especially* independently of it, was correlated with a decreased likelihood of "medical" intervention. Doctors' psychosocial talk had a similar influence, but when controlled for such talk on the part of the patient, that relationship vanished. Were the doctors facilitating patient psychosocial talk? Or were the patients ready and needing to explore their lives, and the doctors ready and willing to listen to them? Whatever it was, these "partly psychosocial" consultations were less likely to result in a referral or a test.

In an interesting, separate study by Salmon and Peters et al. comparing GPs who refused versus accepted training to improve medical management of patients' medically unexplained symptoms, he found that those who refused, who often had denigrating attitudes toward such patients, were already engaging in psychological techniques with them (11). Their behavior belied their statements. They speculated that perhaps these clinicians were more emotionally challenged by such patients, or that they had adopted culturally prevalent attitudes devaluing psychological work in comparison with biomedical work. They made a plea for exploring "how these putative effects of dualism can be overcome."

Models

Psychologists have proposed theories to explain medically unexplained symptoms for the better part of the last century. It is these models to which

Olde Hartman (above) referred when he spoke of the apparent ignorance of clinicians in approaching a patient with MUS. Within the last 20 years, neurobiologists and brain researchers have offered new contributions. The field is complex, in part due to the multiple concepts clinicians describe (hypochondriasis, for instance, is not the same as having a medically unexplained symptom) and evolving. I will attempt here to present information clinicians might find useful when confronted with an actual patient.

Not all medically unexplained symptoms are caused by trauma. A theory which begins to explain them has to encompass those that are and those that are not (and those for which the presence of trauma is unknown). Brown (12) proposes we consider patient vulnerabilities, precipitating events, factors which support continuation of symptoms, and factors which affect such symptoms while they are active. Trauma, Brown feels, is a precipitating factor, as is the witnessing of physical or disease states in others, or educational and cultural influences on a given patient.

Brown's model incorporates the 100_{+} year old theory of Janet, who was trying to explain only the precipitating event of trauma. Janet based his theory on the mental process of dissociation (see Chapter 4). The theory embraces the mental activities of attention, perception, and memory. Traumatic events narrow the focus of attention, so that the person is highly aware of certain aspects of the trauma. However, other experiences of the event are ongoing and recorded in memory but unavailable consciously to the person, and actually outside of their control. However, they can return as sensory events (pain, smells, visual images), affects (fear, sadness), or motor events (tics, freezing). Importantly, since they were recorded without conscious attention, they can appear again without conscious attempt—hence their appearance to this person not as memory but as an invading, unbidden phenomena—understood then as a symptom, or a disease, **not** as a memory. Underneath this is the proposition that there are two different information processing systems—a conscious, "explicit, higher" one, which is disturbed (narrowed) during trauma, and an unconscious, "implicit, lower" one, which continues to function and store memories.

Norman and Shallice's (13) work on the brain localized such an explicit system to the prefrontal cortex. Called the supervisory attentional system (SAS), they proposed that it monitors events and directs behavior in situations where thinking is required—for instance, novelty or stress. The lower-level implicit system, as conceived by Brown based on Shallice et al.'s work, stores memories as postulated by Janet. Its location (in Brown's article) remains unspecified. Just how these two work together is also not laid out, but it is theorized that the activity of the implicit system is what makes these symptoms feel to a patient that the symptoms have nothing to do with their will. The primary activation of the SAS is required to make something feel as if it is under voluntary control.

The SAS may be involved in perpetuating symptoms around trauma or other "precipitating events." Rief and Broadbent (14) have summarized psychological and behavioral mechanisms underlying medically unexplained symptoms. In considering Brown's theory, they note that the SAS may facilitate symptom preservation by focusing attention on the memory traces/symptoms, help-seeking and disease-confirming activities, and awareness of negative affect around symptoms. Thus, the basis of this theory involves perception, modulated by attention and integrated with memory. I would add that other factors that may perpetuate symptoms might be social and interpersonal ones; the responses generated in family, friends, and in ourselves as care providers and our systems.

Other salient and relevant features emerge from Rief and Broadbent's review. They note that patients with medically unexplained symptoms may "catastrophize" their complaints; may attach both medical and psychological explanations to them; tend to pay more attention than average to what signals they are getting from their bodies; are more symptomatic when and if they have a lack of distractions, including physical exercise; and have an increased level of worry about illness in general.

In the realm of behavior, Rief and Broadbent review the literature on alexithymia (the inability to feel one's feelings) which some postulate may underly medically unexplained symptoms (the idea being that if a feeling cannot be felt, it might come out as a physical complaint). Noting the multiplicity of studies and the difficulty of studying feelings that a person does not have, they come to the conclusion that alexithymia is more a precursor (i.e., a patient vulnerability) for mental and psychosomatic disorders in general rather than a specific risk factor (precipitant) for somatization.

Roelofs and Spinhoven (15), reviewing the neurobiology of MUS, discuss the role of the HPA axis and its alterations after trauma. Discussing McEwen's (16) work:

> [T]he individual's response to stress is generated by a network of integrative brain structures involving sub-regions of the hypothalamus... amygdala and periaqueductal gray. These structures receive input from visceral and somatic afferents and from cortical structures, in particular the ventral subdivision of the anterior cingulate cortex and the medial prefrontal... cortices. This integrative network provides outputs to the pituitary and to the pontomedullary nuclei... (which) respectively mediate the neuroendocrine and autonomic output to the body.

There seems to be general agreement that early life trauma induces long-lived and sometimes permanent change in reactivity in this network, such that many (not all) traumatized people have reduced cortisol responsiveness to stress, perhaps mediated by changes in the immune system. People with somatoform disorders share this feature with patients who have mood and anxiety disorders.

What may be more unique in patients with MUS is that structures in the brain that inhibit pain perception, such as the anterior cingulate and the orbitofrontal cortex, may be down-regulated—or sometimes up-regulated—in such patients. Studies with different groups of patients (e.g., with functional bowel disorders) have been contradictory. The best that can be said, perhaps, is that the function of these areas of the brain is changed in such people.

Roelof and Spinhoven sum up this research again by proposing that early trauma, viewed in this lens, may be not just a precipitating factor as above, but also a predisposing factor toward the development of a somatization disorder, both by its effect on the attentional system and the storage of memories, and its effect on the stress response systems of the brain.

Chaos

Stone (17) warns of the potential for "chaos" in a consultation involving medically unexplained symptoms. The chaos, I believe, reflects the internal state of the patient, the internal state of the doctor, or both. The patient is uncomfortable, bewildered, frightened by symptoms. The patient may well possess a story which was also overwhelming, painful, and frightening, often unremembered or even unconscious. The patient often feels shabbily treated by previous practitioners who devalued symptoms that could not fit into a scientific framework, or by friends and relatives who subtly looked down on the diagnosis-less person. The doctor, meanwhile, may be challenged by the patient's non-linear presentation, odd language, or lack of language. "This patient is a poor historian." The doctor may feel stupid, incompetent, or anxious due to the inability to fit the symptoms into a scientific framework. The patient's mien, or unconscious feelings, may be overwhelming or distasteful. Additionally, the doctor may feel guilty about any or all of these reactions. All of these thoughts and feelings swirl, as the two undertake the proscribed dance of diagnosis and treatment. What is not spoken threatens to overpower the work, at any moment.

It is the doctor's job to manage this chaos. This is done, often in reflection and hindsight. With practice, it may improve.

Bonnie

I had 20 minutes with Bonnie some years back. She was a woman in her 40s with morbid obesity, a history of childhood sexual abuse, and the single parent of two pre-adolescent children. She worked as a telephone operator. She participated sporadically in a weight loss program, attending and dropping out of groups, gaining and losing "the same" 20 pounds, and being quite leery of bariatric surgery, which lurks in the background of this program as an option. She came in to discuss her weight progress, which was non-existent. She had recently again begun attending a new group focused on medical weight loss. She had run out of her benefit for the liquid meals, which had helped in the past. She didn't want to know what her weight was. She knew it was up. There was an overall air of hopelessness, futility about her. At the same time, a small smile of triumph played about her lips—as if the weight had won, and she had bet on it all along. I noticed the smile, then quickly began to feel impatient, then dismissive, then angry. Why were we even talking about this? It was clear we were going in circles! Why had I had the idea to have Bonnie come in periodically? I just wanted her to leave. Imperceptibly, Bonnie changed the subject to that of one of her pre-teen's behavior. I didn't notice this until we were there. The son had been an attentive, helpful latency-age child. Now he had begun to have a mind of his own, sometimes acting up in class. He didn't always come right home from school. Bonnie wasn't sure where he was, or what he was doing. There were moments when he was critical of his mother, or mildly defiant. We could talk about this, or... not. Suddenly I felt some of Bonnie's dilemma, and I felt connected to her and our time together, again. How could she parent her pre-adolescent child well, when she herself as a teen had had her boundaries violated, her young womanhood shamed, and her defenses raised to this current, life-threatening level? How could we talk, mother to mother, in a way that could help her manage the anxiety that comes to every parent who watches their child naively face the dangers of the world? Knowing what she knows about what can happen, how can she begin to let go?

In this indirect fashion, perhaps we were circling around some of Bonnie's issues. But we were probably also avoiding something important. I think now about Bonnie's face, her smile. Who was in that smile, so happy that she had yet again failed to break out of her self-defeating eating pattern? I reacted to it as if it were her—and now I see the person of her abuser—a captor, really, who knew he had a trapped victim. I am ashamed now of how easily I too fell into his trap (of feeling irritated with Bonnie and minimizing the work we were trying to do). I'm furious at him, too. My job with Bonnie is to help her reframe her choices, to choose wisely, to gather courage and strength, to offer hope. In a way, also, it is to SEE her—not just her obese body, but the person deep inside. His presence, in her smile, derailed me, and I had not been aware. Perhaps, had I consciously registered the smile's presence, its possible meaning, I could have made use of it. I could have said something like "I can see that you are trying to get yourself back on track again, and yet

I sense there is a part of you that doesn't believe that this will work." Where could we have gone with that?

Is Obesity a Somatization Disorder?

The Adverse Childhood Experiences Study referred to previously (Chapter 6) is a longitudinal study looking at the effect of 18 stressful events potentially occurring in the lives of over 17,000 individuals in Southern California before the age of 18. Eighteen outcome measures of physical, mental, and social health were examined. "ACEs" (childhood stressors) included emotional, physical, and sexual abuse; substance abuse and mental illness in a caregiver; separation/divorce/abuse/incarceration of parents/caregivers. Examples of physical outcomes include sleep disturbances, morbid obesity, substance abuse, multiple somatic symptoms, and disturbances of sexuality. The study is a joint project of Kaiser Permanente and the US Center for Disease Control. The study found strong, graded relationships between the number of ACEs and the likelihood of all 18 outcomes. For instance, individuals with four or more ACEs were 1.9 times more likely than those with none to be morbidly obese, 2.7 times more likely to have multiple somatic symptoms, 5.5 times more likely to be at risk of perpetrating intimate partner violence, and 7.2 times more likely to have the disease of alcoholism.

In a seminal paper resulting from this study, Anda et al. (18) discuss the "convergence" of epidemiologic evidence from their study with emerging evidence from the study of the brain. They review some of the research emerging from the neurosciences, indicating that childhood stressors may permanently alter the developing brain. Changes have been observed in mammalian and human brains in structure and function of the hypothalamic pituitary axis (see above), the hippocampus (early abuse may decrease adult size of this part of the brain, which has a role in learning and memory), and overall neurotrophin production and neuronal survival (children lacking developmentally appropriate experience or exposed to trauma may enter later life with brains fundamentally abnormal in structure and physiology). They tie the anatomic and physiologic evidence to the health and social outcomes mentioned above, strengthening their arguments for a causal relationship, not just an association, between ACEs and adult health. They conclude: "[T]here is a striking convergence of recent findings from the neurosciences with those from a large epidemiologic study of the long-term effects of ACEs which has the potential to open multidisciplinary approaches to studying and improving human well-being. Current practices of medicine and public health are fragmented.... Prevention and remediation of our nation's leading health and social problems is likely to benefit from understanding that many of these problems tend to be co-morbid and may have common origins in the enduring neurodevelopmental consequences of abuse and related adverse experiences during childhood."

Felitti and others co-authored an article (19) reviewing a long-standing treatment experience at Kaiser with obesity. In 1982, they began treating the morbidly obese with prolonged modified fasting, plus a weekly support group, with weight losses of up to 300 pounds. "The striking results perhaps understandably led us to believe that we understood what we were doing. Counterintuitively, some of our most successful patients forced us to realize we were merely in possession of a powerful technology and had no idea what we were doing in other regards. They did this by demonstrating that massive weight loss could precipitate divorce, severe anxiety, and sometimes suicidality. Some patients, sensing these outcomes early, fled their own success in the Program. Surprisingly, our high dropout rate was mainly limited to patients who were *successfully* losing weight (italics his). By contrast, we had other patients who were eating during the Program, routinely denying it, and losing no weight while paying a fairly significant fee, seemingly to accomplish nothing. With these patients, it took some time for us to realize that we were supplying an important support system with our group approach. It turned out that many of our obese patients had no functional support systems at home."

After intensively studying a subset of their very obese patients, they realized that a large number of them grew up with childhood abuse or "dysfunctional households." This finding led to the initiation of the ACE study, as well as to a very different understanding of the disease of obesity. "Ultimately, we learned from our patients that... we are dealing with two core problems:

- The unconscious, compulsive use of food for its psychoactive benefits
- The unrecognized and unspoken *benefits* of obesity."

He goes on to exhort physicians to take such extensive life histories, not to fear doing so, noting that patients often are far more comfortable and relieved discussing them than their physicians (initially at least) are. "Putting it plainly in regard to obesity, we have seen that obesity is not the core problem. Obesity is the marker for the problem and sometimes is a solution. This is a profoundly important realization because none of us expects to cure a problem by treating its symptom." (I would add that we cannot cure a problem by removing its solution either, something Fellitti et. all clearly learned.) He notes that such history-taking will be difficult, both because "polite people" don't discuss such things as rape, incest, and brutality; and also because it's tempting for us, in our ignorance, to label obesity as a "disease"—as if we understood it and because—if we are not obese, or perhaps even if we are—it is difficult to understand how "good" a solution obesity is to a problem that we barely grasp. He also stresses the power of the group experience in exploring the underpinnings of each member's obesity, working on alternate ways of coping with those feelings, and alternate ways of solving the "problem" that harmful life experiences pose.

Felitti et al. worked in the realm of epidemiology and large numbers and have given us extraordinary insights. What does the literature say about the work of the clinician, in the one-on-one?

How We Might Proceed—Part One

"Re-attribution" is one model put forth to help patients and clinicians alike with the mind-body issues that emerge when treating MUS. As I understand it, this framework involves a four-stage process with the patient encompassing a full understanding of the symptoms, an exploration of the patient's psychosocial milieu, the clinician's linking the symptoms timewise or with physiology, and a phase of negotiation. Salmon, Peters et al. explored with a group of patients in the United Kingdom why this model seems to improve patient satisfaction with their health care yet fail to improve outcome (better health) (20). They found that patients were challenged by the complexity of their symptoms (and time allotted to explore them); that they already had "rich psychological narratives" to accompany their symptoms; that they felt their GP had overly simplistic, dualistic ways of looking at symptoms; that they worried therefore that going along with a psychological explanation this time might jeopardize their future biomedical needs. Finally, what the patients seemed to mostly be seeking was support for their self-management.

What emerged as a critical variable in the strength of the relationship, and therefore satisfaction the patient had with their relationship, was the amount of trust the patient had for the physician. Factors that influence patient trust, they noted, "include feeling one's individual experience has been understood and the perceived thoroughness of the evaluation. This is likely to be particularly important in medically unexplained symptoms where individuals recognize that their condition is at the limits of medical knowledge, describe the effort involved in presenting as credible and legitimate, and believe they are taken less seriously than their counterparts with explained symptoms." They made a plea for "increasing GPs' ability to recognize and respond to cues... as important in gaining the trust of... patients." It is possible that the first phase of this model (developing a full understanding of symptoms) is the most important of all.

Waitzkin and Magana (21) have taken the concept of "exploration" further in their work with Central American refugees presenting with symptoms such as weakness, sensory disturbances, headaches, sweating, and hyperventilation. These patients had experienced death threats, rape, and the extermination of loved ones by legal and extralegal forces, in addition to the perils of migration, immigration, and life in a new country, culture, and language. They theorized that undergoing traumatic experience leaves an imprint of a "terrible narrative" which then either disables the person psychologically, or "may (then) be transformed into somatic symptoms.... We would argue that the mechanism by which trauma is transformed into somatic symptoms often involves an incoherence in narrative structure, because of which the traumatic experience cannot be told as a coherent whole." Working when possible with colleagues in psychiatry and social work, these internists and family doctors postulate the importance of the patient's developing a "coherent narrative" as a basis for healing. However, often their patients resist psychological explanations and referral, leaving the family doctors to listen. Often, too, their stories were entwined with the type of chaos referred to by Stone. Thus, they described patients hearing voices from time to time, seeming disembodied from their own stories, and telling disjointed tales of experiences and physical symptoms with no apparent understanding of sequence or meaning. In short, there was much evidence of dissociation (see Chapter 4).

Waitzken et al., almost as an aside, are forced to reshape the term "narrative" to mean not just conventional stories but fragments of them that appear in their research into clinic visits. "In our own prior work on communication in medical encounters, we have found that patients' narratives tend to be interrupted or referred to in passing." This seems to point to a clear need in training especially young clinicians in tolerance for confusion, and in the skills of communication and listening to such stories, difficult as they are.

Waitzkin and Magana discuss the fact that there are many patients with medically unexplained symptoms who may not have experienced recognizable trauma. In advancing their proposal that an "incoherent narrative" waits underneath the somatic symptoms, they note that there is "substantial variability that manifests itself in the connections among trauma, culture and somatization." The fragmentation of the story, for whatever reason, may be what links the "many patients whose physical symptoms cannot be explained by physical disease."

A contribution to treatment emerges near the end of the article as these two writers liken coherent narrative to testimony, and by implication, listeners (clinicians) to culturally sanctioned witnesses. This certainly suggests such a role for a treating clinician. Acknowledging that we lack clarity on optimal treatment, Waitzkin et al. also describe experimenting with the power of structured groups as places to develop more coherence for patients, enable witness to each other, develop "empowered speech," and hopefully come to empowered action in their own lives. (In this regard see the stories of the women in Chapter 6, Peg's husband below, and the treatment groups at Kaiser above.)

Sharon

Sharon is a married, semi-retired human services consultant. Both a mother and grandmother, she spends time with her family and volunteers in art shows, where she often does much of the "grunt work" of getting an exhibition off the ground. She tends to get over-committed. Sharon smoked moderately heavily for 35 years and gave it up with difficulty. She worried about weight gain (which happened). She did not bargain on increased anxiety, which also happened. Despite these undesirable effects, she has never relapsed. She has one or two drinks nightly and has never abused alcohol or drugs.

Sharon's father died fairly young, possibly of aortic stenosis. She worried about dying of heart disease, too. She knew her long history of smoking put her at risk.

After quitting smoking, she began to have an increased intensity of several types of chest pain. Some seem fleeting, some seem related to reflux, but a third type, which she describes as "a tight clamp and achiness" or as "a breath in my throat" or "sharp pains going up both sides under my arms" has been refractory to explanation. Her physical exams and EKGs are always normal. Things escalated some years ago when her brother became terminally ill and died before his time within a period of months. This brother had been involved in some substance abuse. His death was not gentle.

Sharon had a period of intense grief and wondering. During her brother's illness and following it, there was an escalation of her own suffering. She visited several times a year for the chest pain and accompanying fear that something dreadful was going to happen. She was hospitalized for a cardiac workup, which was negative. Then a friend died of coronary disease, and that year there were eight visits for chest pain, including several with an understanding cardiologist. He eventually did a coronary CT to look for calcification, which was utterly benign. He thought things had settled down, but they had not. She continued to visit frequently and to ask me, "what IS this?"

Several years ago, Sharon began to understand and vocalize that she had to "learn not to panic" despite her terror. She continued to visit every couple of months with frightening pain. On one occasion, she came in to tell me that she had realized that if she got overburdened, she was more likely to have pain. She told me, "I was always the child who had to please." She began to say no sometimes to new projects. A few weeks later, she came in saying that now the pain pattern seemed to happen in the middle of the night, out of sleep, and that she was awakening after a nightmare. In the nightmare, men were trying to break into her home, and she felt "trapped and helpless."

This pattern of nighttime terror persisted, and eventually Sharon was again admitted to the hospital, and at the suggestion of cardiology underwent a (negative) cardiac catheterization. She also had an endoscopy, showing minimal esophagitis. She felt "different" after the studies, knowing she had healthy coronaries. There was a six-month reprieve of visits, following which the pains began again, continuing with the pattern of awakening with odd pain, a sense of foreboding, and sometimes the dreams about men breaking into the house and her needing to protect self, children, grandchildren, and feeling helpless. A recent visit followed a memorial service for a friend who had been difficult, and at times violent.

Sharon's story typifies some of the difficulties and ambiguities involved in caring for a person with such a symptom. After a decade, I cannot answer her simple question, "what is wrong?" The specialists can tell her what she does NOT have, at least right now, at least based on symptoms, which offers some "reassurance" but raises other questions. Given her history, the chance of coronary disease and early death is always there, and peers' actual deaths energize these fears in Sharon and in me. Yet her story is highly atypical for coronary disease, or anything else. This is a comfort we can both hold on to. Taking the history EACH TIME, as if each episode is something new, is a vital component of a successful approach. We speak and listen to the words at each encounter, and listen to associations as well, and to new and old patterns. We remain open to physiologic and psycho-physiologic processes. Many times, at the end of a visit, a conclusion is ambiguous, but the anxiety has become manageable. Other times, there's a sense of panic, or a feeling of "I can't handle this anymore." Often, it is hard to know if this feeling is in the patient, the doctor, or both, but it often leads to an expensive "rule out" action (hospitalization, imaging). Following this, there's a temporary calming, but then the process reboots itself. Sharon continues for regular visits, requesting an EKG or needing a soothing visit because of some repetition of nighttime awakening accompanied by pain.

Sharon certainly may fall into the category of someone who lives with a dissociated (implicit) memory, someone who has a dysregulated HPA axis, or a poorly functioning anterior cingulate gyrus. Pain, anxiety, and perhaps features of whatever underlies the symptom have lent the story incoherence. As I listen to and think about her, I have a complex task. I will continue to listen to her story, listen for new organic disease, acknowledge her suffering, join her in her fears, and investigate the unknown. I'll be alert for new stories, and wonder.

Lately, wondering has led to a new part of the story. Sharon has been sharing more about her early family life. When she was eight or nine, her father lost interest in his marriage and began seeing someone else. When her mother found out, she became "hysterical" and was hospitalized on a mental ward for one week for intensive treatment. Sharon and her little brother were told their mother was visiting family. No one spoke of the father's actions. Sharon recalls nothing of how her mother or her family was after her mother returned home. The family remained together for a number of months after the parents had decided on a divorce. The children were not told of this decision either, but Sharon observed shreds of her parent's feelings. Then, her father left "on business" and was gone for months, without explanation. Finally, Sharon's mother, alone with her one morning, asked her, "Do you have any questions?" Straight off, Sharon asked about her parents' relationship. She got the answer that she knew, did not know, and was dreading.

What might I wonder? Does Sharon have other memories for which there are yet no words, only fragments that have not surfaced? What needs in her might be expressed by the pains? Do I actually know all of her "ACEs" in addition to the father's early demise, her family's hiding of their important secrets, the siblings and friends who are violent and involved in self-abusive habits? (and why is this, anyway?) What role should I play in Sharon's exploration of her own fears? Where, now in her life, is she trapped, helpless, unable to escape (and needing to protect others)? Who do the men in her dreams represent? Is this a recall of an actual situation, as it was in Rosita's story (Chapter 6)? I think back to my own training, watching a gifted psychiatrist interviewing a psychotic elderly woman who was hearing men at her door, terrified. He wondered aloud how long it had been since "there was a man at your door?" This was the first time I had seen a doctor connecting the fear and the wish. But how relevant, really, are my own associations to Sharon's life?

Integrating the Knowledge of Abuse into Care

Some research on childhood abuse and the body focuses on prevalence of complaints or described disorders. Thus, there seems to be a higher-than-average incidence of sexual abuse in the histories of those visiting a referral GI practice or presenting to a primary care clinic with irritable bowel symptoms. Other clusters of symptoms have been associated with childhood abuse including gynecologic disorders, pelvic pain, difficulties with parturition, headache, chronic pain, musculoskeletal complaints, and so on.

Research looking at associations is very useful in alerting us to the possibility of childhood sexual abuse as a component of our patient's problem. It doesn't do much for the practicing physician, however, who needs a framework within which to proceed with a complaint. Once we have the idea that a somatization disorder is present, how does this affect our day-to-day work?

Leserman et al. (22) looked at sexual and physical abuse histories in women attending a referral GI practice in North Carolina. Presenting complaints and disorders were not a focus of this study. Of 731 eligible women over a two-year period, 506 agreed to filling out a questionnaire, and among those 506, 239 agreed to return for a full day of interviews and further study. Of the 239, 55% had experienced sexual abuse (childhood and adult), and 48% had experienced physical abuse. Of the other 267, who only filled out the questionnaire, 38% had been sexually abused. Forced sexual touching and rape, as well as physical abuse involving life-threatening force, was associated with significantly more non-GI symptoms such as headache, backache, and fatigue, and also with more psychological distress and functional disability. Rape and force, but not less invasive abuse, were associated with more current pain, disability, and lifetime surgeries. In sub-analyses, it seemed that either one or many episodes of abuse resulted in the same decline in health status. In this study, the timing of first abuse (before or after the age of 14) did not affect the magnitude of poor outcome. Leserman and her colleagues noted that of those patients who had a history of abuse, only 17% of the gastroenterologists being referred these patients "acknowledged" discussing this history with the patients. She concludes that in light of the relationship between abuse and negative health outcomes, "it is reasonable that asking about present and past abuse become an essential part of history-taking in medical practice, and that referral for psychological services be made available when appropriate."

Douglas Drossman (23,24), in his presidential address to the American Psychosomatic Society in 1998, explored how George Engel's biopsychosocial model might apply in understanding the varying courses of illness and disease seen in several patients with GI disturbance. He challenges the Cartesian dualism still present in medicine (mind **or** body) by probing more deeply into our understanding of varying symptoms and outcomes of patients with GERD, functional bowel disease, and Crohn's disease. He integrates findings from neurophysiology and helps us think about psychosocial history and effects of the brain, being willing to understand functional disease as a disease of brain and organ. He calls attention to a study of "1000 patients with inflammatory bowel disease, (in which) the frequency of physician visits was predicted primarily by psychosocial factors, whereas disease activity and symptom ratings were not predictive of such visits." He concludes with a call for research in a broad variety of areas, including psychoimmunology, pharmacology with drugs targeted toward gut AND brain, cross-cultural research, and research on the patient–doctor relationship, among others. He also states, "more work is needed to teach health care professionals and the public about the legitimacy of psychosocial factors in medical illness and patient care."

The literature confirms our need to have a high index of suspicion about abuse in certain circumstances. Once we are convinced of the "legitimacy of psychosocial concerns" (see the first incident in this chapter)—what do we then know, and do? As generalists, we may refer some of our patients for psychological work; but many will stick with us for the majority of their concerns. In other words, much of the disease and illness which prior mistreatment causes will be played out in the theatre of the body, with the patient and the clinician as participant-observers or actors. Much of whatever healing occurs may need to happen within the patient, with the primary caregiver as midwife, until society (and that includes all of us) comes to terms with its shameful permission for and ignorance of the abuse and neglect of its young people—on battlegrounds, in bedrooms, on the streets, and in schools and training programs of all kinds.

Peg

Peg came for general medical care decades ago. At that point she had been married for some time and had four adolescent children. Both she and her husband worked in human services. She had a history of irritable bowel syndrome, hypertension, and a goiter, possibly due to Hashimoto's disease. She had had, before I met her, multiple surgical procedures—a urethral dilatation, cholecystectomy, two oophorectomies (one partial, for dermoids), and an appendectomy. She'd had Bell's palsy twice. She had had lifelong oligomenorrhea and been fertile only with the use of steroid hormones, she said.

Within a few years of starting to work together, Peg developed diabetes mellitus. She had a strong family history of it, and she was 80 pounds overweight. To date, her weight has fluctuated within a 30-pound range, which is 70 to 100 pounds or so overweight.

Early in our work together, Peg disclosed her father's mental illness and the fact that he had sexually assaulted her during her teen years. Her mother was alcoholic. She was a middle child of a large family, of whom one has been psychotic since giving birth, and, by the time Peg reached 60, several other sibs had died.

Both she and her husband were hard and honest workers, and both were morbidly obese. They were happily married. Their children all grew up, married happily, and became reliable workers as well.

Over the years, Peg has usually seen me frequently, as often as once or twice a month, with four or five phone calls per year in between. One might surmise she would be seen rather regularly for "control" of diabetes and hypertension and associated issues. However, her blood pressure has always been in excellent control on a small amount of medication despite her weight, requiring almost no input from either of us. Her diabetic control seems to have eluded both of us. For a while, she saw a local endocrinologist who stopped meds I started because of GI side effects—although years later she tolerated the same drugs with no problem. She stopped seeing the specialist around the time she began on insulin, of which she was "petrified," thinking that if she started injecting, she'd develop middle of the night hypoglycemia and die (she was not particularly afraid of using syringes or needles, and she really liked the insulin pen). She rarely called in when asked to while I tried to adjust insulin, and would go for months without contact around this issue. Her glycohemoglobin was at its worst the year after beginning insulin and was at its best when her weight was at its worst. I worked with her on starting a sliding scale and ultra-short acting insulin, and she gave the Humalog away to someone else. I did not find that out for a year. Despite careful explanation, she had taken her first dose one evening before going out to dinner, then been kept waiting by the restaurant for an hour and had a frightening hypoglycemic spell right in public. At her wits end, she gave the vial away (without calling at all). She has never been able to keep off a meaningful amount of weight. So it has gone.

Instead, I saw Peg episodically for complaints that were mostly short-lived, about which she was very anxious and needed immediate reassurance. One year, I saw her 19 times for right-sided abdominal pain (present on and off for many years), nausea, neck pain, chest pain, back pain, headache, worry about a long-standing axillary lipoma which was not changing, a choking sensation, and a tingling trapezius muscle. Notably, most of these issues were accompanied by few physical findings, a sense of impending doom, and rapid resolution once we had checked things out. Visits would end with a sense of expressed relief and gratitude, and also with some humor, one of Peg's strengths. The underlying joke: here we are again. However, there was little memory or insight from one visit to the next. Severe temporal pain would bring her in after two visits for abdominal pain, without reference to what had been going on last month. In addition, each episode of abdominal pain was presented as the first, though they'd been going on for years.

The freshness and anxiety were communicable; it was as hard for me to remember that Peg had symptoms consistent with irritable bowel syndrome as it was for me to try to keep the threads of her diabetes straight.

Slowly, several other themes emerged. During the year when she visited most, she was also in a very difficult work situation. She had been promoted against the will of an immediate supervisor, as well as a co-worker (a friend of the supervisor's) who wanted the job. She was harassed mercilessly by them, and a few months later accepted a "demotion," continuing to feel humiliated by these two. She was made the butt of jokes by both of them. Within weeks of the demotion, she was briefly hospitalized for chest pain. The pain was highly atypical of coronary disease, and the history was not revealed to the ER staff; she had "coronary risk factors" and was admitted and "ruled out." With the encouragement of her husband, she filed harassment charges; her documentation somehow got "lost." I started her on an antidepressant and referred her to a social worker, whom she saw sporadically and whom she felt helped her. At one point she told me, when coming in complaining that she felt intolerable throat tension and "choking," that she felt "paralyzed by work." The social worker recommended a leave, which she did not take. Miraculously, both of these supervisors retired at the end of the year; Peg again applied for the more senior job—and was chosen. Her new boss was not an easy person, but someone who was straightforward and fair, and Peg thought she could deal with her.

Peg's increased symptoms developed in the context of humiliation, shame, the undermining of her personal power. Her time with the social worker likely provided her with a valuable witness and the creation of strategies and options. Her physical symptoms and the emotions they aroused—fear of annihilation, dread—can be seen as part of this picture. Our work together included looking and palpating the dreaded object, re-naming it as something benign, and then sometimes placing the whole incident in perspective—shared laughter, "Wasn't this silly," on the part of Peg. Her husband, who often brought her, once told me, "You two are more like sisters than anything else."

For several years after beginning antidepressants, Peg complained of lack of sexual desire. She stated that she and her husband had had a mutually enjoyable sex life, but at around the time of the above (which was also the year of her menopause), she had lost interest. She intermittently worried about the effect on her husband and on their relationship. We adjusted medications and actually ended up trying four of them in an effort to get around this. Recently she complained that actually, her lack of interest had another component. Her husband (who had always been pleasing to her) "always needed to be in command" and this was now an annoyance. She was unsure how to proceed. How should she now handle herself, how should she talk to him, could sex really be any other way? She was not sure she wanted to undertake that whole conversation.

Finally, during this same year, Peg's husband retired. This sparked thoughts of retirement in her, which worried her—wondering how they would get by, wondering if she should do the same, and so on. Meanwhile her husband (also a patient) began to pursue a second career as a "high school teacher" as he put it. He made himself available to local high schools to talk about his military experience in Vietnam, the nightmares he has had for years about combat, and the truth as he saw it about US involvement overseas. He had also begun to attend the new (due to Iraq/Afghanistan casualties and public perceptions) PTSD groups at the local VA, and he now meets weekly there to discuss his own flashbacks and symptoms with other Vietnam veterans. He had barely alluded to them in the 20 or so years I have known him. When he describes them to me now, this laconic working-class man is moved to tears. He is also more obese than ever. But he is aware that what he has to say is of value to young people, whether they know it or not.

How We Might Proceed—Part Two

Stone (25,26,27) has written several papers studying effective generalists' approaches to patients with medically unexplained symptoms. Using grounded theory, a qualitative approach, she spoke with generalists in Australia, both experienced and novice, to understand the basis for successful management. Tellingly, and as an aside, she spoke of the need to gain the trust of the registrars (novices) before they would tell her how they thought and felt, because of the effects both of dualistic training (body or mind) and of harsh training experiences:

> I had a number of them share their stories of hospital-based learning, where questions were discouraged, support was elusive and at times they faced painful, challenging experiences alone without an opportunity to debrief. In the interviews, I found I needed to spend a lot of time developing rapport and demonstrating empathy, validating the participant's experience before they were prepared to be open and honest about their thinking, and importantly, their feelings. Many did not expect their thinking to be valued and needed reassurance, both explicit and implicit, before they were prepared to be open about their clinical practice (26).

Is there any wonder that it takes beginning practitioners some time to explore what might work with patients who are feeling the same thing? Is medical training, for some, its own variety of abuse and neglect of the young?

Stone found that novices and experienced practitioners alike articulated several effective behaviors. They were:

1. Validate the patient's suffering. Accept that the symptoms are real and cause real distress. Acknowledge the frustration caused to date and ongoing by the lack of an understanding. Assume the yoke of responsibility. One young doctor stated, "We are the only ones who may have some hope of actually seeing that there is a physical component that we actually have to manage and at the same time being accessible, inquiring, encouraging and supportive of the psychological walk, whether or not that's with another health professional, this is the only place where the body and mind actually become one. And if that's not our job then I don't know whose job it is." Another said, "The patient's just an inconvenient accompaniment to the disease in the hospital, but it's the other way around in the community" (17).

2. Give the illness a name. In our culture, people suffering without a label suffer blame and shame. Use the patient's words, if possible, with the caveats below.
3. Avoid thought-labels which dismiss the patient, both by self and consultants, such as "borderline personality disorder" "large demanding blob" etc. At the same time try to broaden the agenda of treatment to include social and psychological strategies.
4. Try to avoid over-referral, over-medicalization, and the tendency for a cascade of specialists, while at the same time keeping an eye out for new, perhaps more physiologically understood diseases. The situation is dynamic, and changes with time. Some doctors need to alternate the broader (Engel's biopsychosocial) approach with a more strictly medical one. "You sort of ... pop your head up ... you put the periscope up now and then to see if there is a way, there is an island nearby or a way out, otherwise you're just there with the patient travelling with them" (26).

Speaking from my own experience, I feel honored, mostly, and burdened, sometimes, by the "Pegs" in my practice, their trust in me and our ability to work through the times when they fear for their lives. There are times when I have to be more responsive on the telephone than I am sometimes really wanting to be. It helps me to remember that to a Peg, this is a life and death situation, just as her teenage experiences with her father raping her were.

I recommend a steady hand, and orderly record keeping, in dealing with the many anxious complaints of a Peg. They will keep her health care costs and unnecessary health care experiences down. Fear and dread can be contagious and disorienting. Once we are floating in it, we're just as lost as the patient was, and now still is. It takes mental strength to realize we've lost our moorings, and we have to make our prior work clear to ourselves so we can find it again.

I am proud of the fact that Peg had had five abdominal and pelvic surgeries before she met me, but only one (for an infected Bartholin's cyst) since we met.

I'm happy for Peg that she chose a husband who understands her struggles to be similar to his own and who can recognize those in me ("you two are like sisters"). I regret not having done the same sleuthing with her husband as I have done with her. On the other hand, he has been far more elusive, less seeking of care until recently.

I wish health care policy and program directors were as honest as Felitti et al. are about their successes and failures and what drives them, and as persistent. I want for Peg to have a "post-combat" support group like her husband does, and for both of them to have it at least weekly; for it to be affordable, and for as long as they need it; to realize a new relationship with food and body size. I am convinced they both have within themselves, with proper guidance, the wisdom to know the truth and literally reshape themselves. Though both are "candidates" for bariatric surgery, I do not believe that is the only answer for either one. I am not sure what approach would work with "somatizers" to, for instance, begin to link and tolerate some of the emotions they feel in their body; to overcome impulsive behavior; to deal with perceived life threats, to overcome early worries of survival that are based in reality. I imagine this to be a long-term endeavor, and meanwhile, coming to the clinician with physical symptoms and attendant powerful emotions will continue to be an unconscious strategy employed by many, one for which we must be prepared.

References

1. Kroenke K and Mangelsdorff AD, "Common symptoms in ambulatory care: incidence, evaluation, therapy and outcome," *American Journal of Medicine* 86(3): 262–266, 1989. Quoted in Edwards TM et al., "The treatment of patients with medically unexplained symptoms in primary care: a review of the literature," *Mental Health in Family Medicine* 7(4): 209–221, 2010.
2. Stone L, "Blame, shame and hopelessness: medically unexplained symptoms and the 'heartsink' experience," *Australian Family Physician* 2014, April; 43 (4), 191–195.
3. Singh BS, "Managing somatoform disorders," *Medical Journal of Australia* 1998: 568–572, as quoted in Stone L and Clarke DM, "Somatising disorders, untangling the pathology," *Australian Family Physician* 36 (3), 234–239, 2007.
4. Stone L and Clarke DM, "Somatising disorders, untangling the pathology," *Australian Family Physician* 36(3): 234, 2007.
5. Cassell EJ, *The Nature of Suffering and the Goals of Medicine*, 2nd edition, Oxford University Press, 2004.
6. Salmon P, Humphris G, Ring A, Davies J, and Dowrick C, "Primary care consultations about medically unexplained symptoms: patient presentations and doctor responses that influence the probability of somatic intervention," *Psychosomatic Medicine* 69: 571–577, 2007.
7. Peters S, et al., "What do patients choose to tell their doctors? Qualitative analysis of potential barriers to reattributing medically unexplained symptoms," *Journal of General Internal Medicine*, 24(4): 443–449, 2008.
8. Epstein R, Shields C, Meldrum S, Fiscella K, Carroll, K, Carney P, and Duberstein P, "Physicians' responses to patients' medically unexplained symptoms," *Psychosomatic Medicine* 68: 269–276, 2006.
9. Olde Hartman TC, Hassink-Franke LJ, Lucassen PL, van Spaendonck KP, van Weel C, "Explanation and relations. How do general practitioners deal with patients with persistent medically unexplained symptoms: a focus group study," *BMC Family Practice*10: 68, 2009. doi:10.1186/1471-2296-10-68.
10. Salmon, H, et al., "Primary care consultations about medically unexplained symptoms," 2007.
11. Salmon P, Peters S, Clifford R, Iredale W, Gask L, Rogers A, et al., "Why do general practitioners decline training to improve management of medically unexplained symptoms?" *Journal of General Internal Medicine* 22: 565–571, 2007.

12. Brown RJ, "Psychological mechanisms of medically unexplained symptoms; an integrative conceptual model," *Psychological Bulletin* 130: 793–812, 2004.
13. Norman DA and Shallice T, "Attention to action: willed and automatic control of behavior," in David RJ et al. (eds.) *Consciousness and Self-Regulation: Vol. 4, Advances in Research and Theory*, pp. 1–18, 1986.
14. Rief W and Broadbent E, "Explaining medically unexplained symptoms-models and mechanisms," *Clinical Psychology Review* 27: 821–841, 2007.
15. Roelofs K and Spinhoven P, "Trauma and medically unexplained symptoms: Towards an integration of cognitive and neuro-biological accounts," *Clinical Psychology Review* 27: 798–820, 2007.
16. McEwen, BS, Protective and damaging effects of stress mediators, *The New England Journal of Medicine* 338: 171–179, 1998.
17. Stone L, Reframing chaos: a qualitative study of GPs managing patients with medically unexplained symptoms, *Australian Family Physician* 42(7): 501–512, 2013.
18. Anda R, Felitti V, Bremner JD, Walker J, Whitfield C, Perry B, et al., "The enduring effects of abuse and related adverse experiences in childhood," *European Archives of Psychiatry and Clinical Neuroscience* 256: 174–186, 2006.
19. Felitti V, Jakstis K, Pepper V, and Ray A, "Obesity: problem, solution, or both?" *The Permanente Journal* 14(1): 24–30, 2010.
20. Salmon, Peters, et al., "Why do general practitioners decline training," *Journal of General Internal Medicine* 22: 565–571, 2007.
21. Waitzkin H and Magana H, "The black box in somatization: unexplained physical symptoms, culture, and narratives of trauma," *Social Science &Medicine* 45(6): 811–825, 1997.
22. Leserman J, Drossman D, Li Z, Toomey T, Nachman G, Glogau K, "Sexual and physical abuse history in gastroenterology practice: how types of abuse impact health status," *Psychosomatic Medicine* 58: 4–15, 1996.
23. Drossman DA, Talley NJ, Leserman J, Olden KW, Barreiro MA, "Sexual and physical abuse and gastrointestinal illness: review and recommendations," *Annals of Internal Medicine* 123: 782–794, 1995.
24. Drossman DA, Presidential address: Gastrointestinal illness and the biopsychosocial model," *Psychosomatic Medicine* 60: 258–267, 1998.
25. Stone L, "Somatising disorders, untangling the pathology," *Australian Family Physician* 36: 234–239, 2007.
26. Stone L, "Making sense of medically unexplained symptoms in general practice: a grounded theory study of supervisors and registrars in general practice," *Mental Health in Family Medicine* 10(2): 101–111, 2013.
27. Stone L, "Managing the consultation with patients with medically unexplained symptoms: a grounded theory study of supervisors and registrars in general practice," *BMC Family Practice*15: 192. 2014. doi:10.1186/s12875-014-0192-7.

8
The Doctor–Patient Relationship

I did not know what to say, my mouth
had no way
with names
my eyes were blind,
and something started in my soul,
fever or forgotten wings,
and I made my own way,
deciphering
that fire,
and I wrote the first faint line,
faint, without substance, pure
nonsense,
pure wisdom
of someone who knows nothing . . .

—*Pablo Neruda* **(1)**

Introduction

No book about the treatment of adults who have survived trauma would be complete without a discussion of the nature of the journey undertaken together by patient and doctor—the ongoing, unfolding relationship in which treatment rests. Although every such relationship is unique, certain themes may emerge while working with adults traumatized in childhood. Doctors and other providers who are charged with "managing" such relationships, as well as experiencing them and using them for the patient's benefit, are best served by understanding some parameters ahead of time. In addition, an enjoyment of the varied texture of such relationships is the basis, the ground on which satisfaction in general medicine exists. Past trauma can disrupt that; or it can be understood and harnessed in a way that helps and heals, sometimes all parties involved.

Perspectives on the Relationship with a Trauma Survivor

Thirty years ago, Elaine Alpert set out some thoughts on physician conduct with trauma survivors. Her seminal 1995 article focused on the treatment of women experiencing domestic violence, but her advice is germane to our subject here (2). She noted that "many patients do not believe their physician knows about the issue, would know what to do, or even cares about (domestic violence)." Other barriers to a full treatment relationship cited by Alpert include victims' shame, fears about confidentiality, and a sense that the issue is out of bounds for a medical encounter. Perhaps most telling, "subtle and usually unintentional victim-blaming statements, minimization, and denial on the part of some health care providers could reinforce the patient's sense of shame, humiliation and responsibility about the violence." She argued for routinizing inquiries about violence and following through, "using an open-ended query format, with the physician maintaining a compassionate, non-judgmental stance."

Many writers other than Alpert emphasize the importance of suspension of judgment on the part of the clinician. Notably, however, they do not tell us how to inculcate such an attitude. We have all matured in a society which both glorifies and shudders openly at violence yet often ignores its effects. Medical education has had little to do, to date, with helping students understand this dialectic. It is to be expected that every clinician, therefore, brings his own history, assumptions, and reactions to the problem, which then colors each encounter he has with a patient. "The physician should never ask questions or make statements that reinforce the patient's sense of shame, humiliation, blame, powerlessness, and failure," says Alpert. She is to be commended for setting the bar high, and correctly in these situations. I think it is unrealistic, however, to expect that we will all effortlessly meet these standards. Rather, we need help learning and correcting our inevitable missteps along the way.

The milieu in which children experience abuse, and its effects on the expectations adults then bring to treatment relationships, is explored by Alaggia. She interviewed 40 adult male and female survivors of child sexual abuse (3). Alaggia was especially interested in what discouraged or prevented children from seeking help after trauma. We can predict that at the very least, patients will bring the imprint of these experiences to their encounters with providers. Her interviewees had experienced, as children:

- Confusion as they viewed sexualized advertisements and media involving young teens.

- Messages that men should never be victims.
- Messages that men should never appear to be homosexual.
- An attitude that children were not to speak out.
- A reality that if they as children did speak up, they were often blamed.
- Insensitivity on the part of those to whom they did speak.
- Being told that they themselves should put a stop to the abuse, if they really did not want it.
- A reality that if they did tell, adults acted to preserve the status quo because of financial dependence of the parent or the social prominence of the abuser, the child's family, or both.
- Physical harm to themselves by family members, who accused them of lying.
- Physician bias: "Well that's not sexual assault, you were old enough (at 13 or 14). You probably enjoyed it, you know. You girls in those countries enjoy those things anyway, that's not sexual assault."

Alaggia suggested that clinicians review with adult clients all their attempts to tell, responses they received, and personal consequences of telling. I think this is a good suggestion, as it will help the current adult victim–clinician duo explore together the patient's experience of the "other." It will also serve as a review, for the clinician, of some of the many realities and pitfalls for her as she brings her own knowledge, experience, and attitudes to the problems the patient may be facing now. Finally, Alaggia suggests that we in medicine could do much more to promote primary prevention and secondary awareness of child abuse, including interactions with the media, education, and justice systems of our current society.

Writing for family physicians, Bala outlines the continuity between adult survivors' presenting symptoms and what she terms the "child sexual abuse accommodation syndrome," as outlined by Summit (4). Emphasizing that adult symptoms can be due to patients' learned coping mechanisms in dealing with the abuse, she outlines some of those symptoms and mechanisms, discussed in this volume in previous chapters (PTSD, self-harm, dissociative disorders, problems experienced in the body). She describes the interpersonal realities that were living features of abuse for the patient, including secrecy, enforced silence, helplessness, accommodation to escalating demands, realization of betrayal by the trusted adult, self-blame, and the conflicted processes involved in disclosure described in previous paragraphs. In addition to symptoms or syndromes, the patient understandably may have great difficulty with trust, interpersonal boundaries, recognition of danger to herself, difficulty with following the rules of the office or clinic, disorganization of behavior or history, and the like. She advocates for physician awareness, a low index of suspicion for prior abuse when such symptoms or behavior are encountered, and an early identification of "this dynamic (to) ensure that the patient is not punished or reabused for her behavior, but rather . . . encouraged to recognize, understand, and change it." I would add that this latter process is one that may take years, just like any of the other behavioral changes we set in front of our patients or ourselves.

Bala encourages providers to develop their own questions about abuse, stressing that what is most important is "the tone of caring, respect and validation. . . . Patients should feel heard and believed. Physicians must convey the clear belief that the abuse was not their fault. Physicians can provide information about the widespread extent of sexual abuse of children and common long-term effects, which could include the patient's symptoms. Physicians might express the belief that the patient's survival thus far reflects her strength and courage, and that her symptoms should be viewed as the vestiges of the survival skills she learned as a child."

Some doctors may have difficulty with some aspects of this behavior asked of them. To be hoped for is that beneath the tone of caring and respect is the reality of caring and respect. Yet all of us have biases. It has been shown that in general (5) men consider trauma survivors less credible than do women; that older victims (teens) are considered less credible than younger ones; and that victims of family members and friends are less credible than victims of strangers.

We need to step outside ourselves and think about our own socialization. For many men, being a victim means losing one's manhood. Most of us forget that over two-thirds of abusers ARE family members, friends, dates. In the face of teen assertions of independence and physical growth, it is easy to forget that teens are still children, lacking the knowledge, power, and resources of adulthood. For providers who are themselves survivors of abuse, patient survivors will activate their own memories and healing, at whatever stage that healing is. For providers who are not, the stark realities of what happened may set in motion normal but powerful forces to forget. As Judith Herman wrote in her groundbreaking book: "The ordinary response to atrocities is to banish them from consciousness. Certain violations of the social compact are too terrible to utter aloud; this is the meaning of the word unspeakable" (6). It will be a struggle for many providers to remember what they have been told by abused patients and to invest it with the importance it has for the patient and for the work of doctor and patient together. For others, the challenge will be to develop the strength and compassion to return to the work again, again, and again. This engagement, however successful, builds the foundation for deserved trust.

Strength is particularly needed when patients are angry. Their anger may be directed at participants in the original scenario. But it often spills over into rage at society, facets of society, men. It is close to the surface when something happens which triggers reminders of the original abuse situation, including unintended slights by providers. It can be enormous and seemingly out of proportion. It can also be projected so that the patient is ready to feel hated or hates her- or himself. Such a person becomes depressed and/or self-destructive (see Chapter 6). Often such patients can't connect the dots, cannot recognize or feel their own anger, cannot place it where it belongs, and when it comes out, feel it is unmanageable. They are frightened to own it, frightened of what it can do. Often anger is underneath whatever brought the patient in. Here the challenge for the doctor will be to remember where it originates, to name it, to help the patient manage it—and to do all this while owning his own role in setting it off, if there is any, without being overcome by guilt, rage, or shame himself. The doctor also cannot, out of his own discomfort, minimize or ignore the anger. It is there for an excellent reason—just not yet processed (7).

Finally, we come to the concept of "enactments." Writing for psychotherapists, Plakun (8) delineates the concepts of transference, countertransference, projective identification, and enactment as historically developed over the last 110 years. Plakun argues that scenarios which replicate in the patient's mind their prior abuse will of necessity need to develop in the course of treatment, though they will also be feared by them. These scenarios will then be invested with specific meaning from the clinician's history and guide the physician's response to them, creating a mutually invested interpersonal drama. These, Plakun states, are inevitable, uncomfortable, and emotion-filled for all involved. They may feel like failures and dead ends; they are the embodiments of the patients' dilemmas. Yet they are also golden opportunities for the patient to understand a new way of being, if the doctor can see into herself, envisioning her own stake in maintaining the status quo.

A crude enactment occurs daily in medicine if, when patients come to us with medically unexplained symptoms (Chapter 7) we react with ignorance, rejection, confusion, or referral, and reach no further understanding on what might be being communicated. It is also reflected in the failure of medical science to explore this domain of physical reality, the failure of medical schools to teach it, and the failure of funding agencies to underwrite understanding. Those who have guided our present levels of knowledge are in essence abandoning patients' suffering, just as did the parent and the neighborhood who suspected but did not act as the child was being abused. When, on an individual level, we dismiss rather than are curious and validating—because we are threatened, confused, or numb and don't like it, and don't want to admit it—we are doing the same thing. The enormous growth seen in alternative medicine is perhaps a testament to this failure of integration on the part of organized medicine.

On a more personal level, patients with abuse histories will come to us, as anyone else does, ready to weave together their life story—their history, their important people, their bodies—into their story with us. For some patients we are parent figures; for some we are siblings, authority figures, teachers, admired sons, and so on. There is a likelihood that for a patient with a childhood abuse history, we will be an abuser, a victim, a bystander, or an imagined rescuer. What Plakun is pointing out is that how our own story intersects with that of the patient determines how we "enact" the patient's stories (and our own). Furthermore, it is the doctor's job to "catch" both "actors" in the act: to realize what is happening and to speak it in service of the patient's recovery. Finally, I would point out that at different times we may be seen, and therefore treated, differently—we may be victimized by the patient one moment, or one year, and the next, experienced as an abuser—or invited to abuse. We may be idealized one day and dreaded or reviled the next. Our own stories, moreover, invite us to step into these different roles with meaning for ourselves.

The work of a psychoanalyst and that of an internist may at first seem many miles apart. However, if we believe in the model of relationship-centered care, we find many similarities. In such care, as conceptualized in internal medicine, the relationship is not the vehicle of treatment, it IS the treatment. For many individuals, the medical relationship carries some of the weight in a patient's mind that a therapy relationship might.

More to the point, working with any patient creates scenarios in which we must live. Working with an abuse survivor creates certain predictable enactments that will trip us up if we are unwary or unaware. We can't victimize, rescue, or ignore the patient; nor can we let this happen to us. We need to set the rules for straightforwardness and caring, and then hold ourselves and the patient to them. When we stray—as both patient and doctor will—we need to notice, to be honest with ourselves and with our patients, and we need to learn and help the patient learn from our and her mistakes. This is the meaning of professionalism.

We are coming to a time in which we have a richer understanding of the nature of human relationships in general, and the doctor–patient relationship in particular. Such an understanding has begun to creep into the training of medical professionals; it has generally lagged biomedical training in detail, richness, and transmission of skill. Seasoned generalists know many features of this in their bones, but the principles and nuances bear repeating here. Suchman (9) has provided a theoretical basis for relationship-centered care in complexity theory, in which the relationship is seen to be both self-organizing and capable of new directions, in which a small stimulus from one party may lead to great long-term change in one or the other, and in which there is continuous meaning-making in everyday patterns. Adler has stressed the fundamental requirement for empathy and discussed its neurobiology. He states, "While biopsychosocial responsiveness between patients and physicians is reciprocal and mutual, it is not symmetrical because patients and society grant clinicians the responsibility to focus attention and treat biological and psychological aspects of a patient's disease. . . . The physician's use of empathy warrants consideration as a clinical procedure because it uses 'emotional resonance' to achieve skilled communicative attunement that produces a neurobiological intervention" (10). He stresses the positive effects of empathic attunement on both doctor and patient, buffering stress for the ill patient and creating a sense of mastery and joy for the doctor.

"Joy" may seem too strong a word in today's era of clinical guidelines, computerized decision support, and time limitations. That's what these writers are talking about, however. Egnew stresses the role of the physician as a healer, helping the patient to accept, transcend, and make sense of his suffering using empathic skills (11). "Because healing is a process, the metamorphosis of the role of doctor to healer is the change from doer to helper, from expert problem solver and fixer to servant and companion, an accompanier on the healing journey. . . . The change from expert-doer to servant-accompanier requires that physicians attend to how they *are* with patients as much as what they *do* for them." (pp. 172–173) I underscore what Egnew is saying. I believe, however, that the expert health practitioner must be capable of both and be able to switch back and forth as needed. For every patient, there are times when we must "do," and others—many others—where we must simply "be," or "be there." Our trauma patients, certainly, need both sides of us (see the story of Elora, Chapter 3).

Angela

Angela's story touches on some of the themes mentioned above and in Chapter 7, including medically unexplained symptoms, the gradual but targeted questioning about abuse issues, and the development of trust. Her medical path included what we might call an enactment, the naming of which led to a richer understanding and reduced anxiety on the part of the patient, myself, and a treating specialist.

Her first visits were to the practice's physician assistant, for upper respiratory complaints, then blood pressure management. Blood pressure had been labile. At her first "complete" exam with me, she revealed she was trying to cut back on cigarettes and on salty foods, as part of her attempt to control blood pressure. Her mother had just been diagnosed with breast cancer. She had gone to work after high school, never attended college, married at 26. The couple had been infertile, and she had had laparoscopic surgery for endometriosis. She eventually had a hysterectomy at a relatively young age. She had been on hormone replacement since that time. She and her husband had adopted and raised a little girl as an infant. Their daughter had just left home for undergraduate school. This was her only child. She had done clerical work, but during her daughter's adolescence had found a new career in the arts and "loved" it. Family history revealed that she hadn't been in touch with her father for over 10 years. He had "left the family" when she was eight years old. There were three younger sibs. There was a strong family history of cancer—breast, ovary.

The next couple of visits centered on blood pressure control and smoking cessation. A year later, she came for "groin pain" with no obvious pathology; it began out of the blue, and went away.

Some time later, Angela came in for general checkup, "depressed and unmotivated." Her daughter, who had seemed to need her during her first year away from home, was getting much more self-sufficient. She had quit exercising, was drinking more, and had gained weight. I took my cue from the seeming grief and anger over her daughter's departure and asked about the her own experience of being mothered. She said felt she was neglected "somewhat," and her mother was emotionally distant. Angela had ended up caring for her mother during the years when she normally would have gone to college. She was also mourning her infertility once again. Four years prior, she and her husband had entered marital counseling. That therapist encouraged her to seek individual counseling because the therapist suspected childhood sexual abuse. Angela agreed, and during this further treatment she recalled "an incident" with her father when she was eight—shortly before he left home. She had later confronted father about why he had left, and said he was "evasive." After two visits with him, she felt she would not be able to get any further with him and didn't bring up specific issues.

I have no more notes on this discussion. Apparently, I did not press the patient on what she recalled happening with her dad; whether there were other times before or later; whether she had told her mother, and what might have happened when she did. All of these questions could have been potentially useful, or might better have waited for another time. Much had been revealed. To a simple association regarding mother/daughter relationships had come much which might be at the root of the current depression, overeating, and alcohol use. It was all worth noting; we also had a physical exam and practical tasks at hand.

Two mundane visits followed, one for a sinus infection and another to discuss whether blood pressure needed treatment.

A year later, at her annual exam—Angela's mood was better. She felt much "calmer" about the daughter's increasing maturity. The daughter had a boyfriend, had traveled some, and was adjusting well at college. She realized that "it didn't hit me 'til she was a sophomore." She was still smoking, still not ready to quit. She thought her gynecologist felt something wrong with her right breast. We had those notes to review, and they did not indicate a problem. I was concerned by this innuendo, given her family history. Careful exam revealed nothing; the subsequent mammogram was normal also. Despite all this, the concern (medically unexplained symptom?) proved to be prescient. We did start her on anti-hypertensives during this visit.

Later that year she consulted me about issues with her daughter's health; the daughter might need spine surgery. Angela felt her daughter's previous doctors had not cared well for her and was concerned that the right one be found now. I was able to help her find a suitable specialist. Her blood pressure had responded to meds.

At her next annual exam, worries about her daughter were much less. The decision had been made not to operate at all on the daughter—or at least not for a long while. Angela's breast concerns had abated. She wanted, however, to stay on post-menopausal hormone therapy, even after we discussed the risks. She had been avoiding colon cancer screening for several years despite our scheduling it for her.

A year later, Angela's mother was "going strong" despite her prior breast cancer, in her ninth decade. The father had recently died. Angela had not had contact with him in many years. Her blood pressure was not ideal, was high normal. She was still avoiding colonoscopy. She appeared "buoyant." The daughter was living in New York and had broken up with a wealthy boyfriend, much to Angela's relief. Later that year, eight days after 9/11/2001, she visited me simply to assure us both that her daughter had been unscathed.

The following year, she lacerated a toe dropping pruning shears on them and required operative repair. Her husband called to make sure they were seeing the "right" foot surgeon. Eventually, they settled on the man who was covered by their insurance, though his office neighborhood bothered her. They were delighted with the results. She finally had a colonoscopy (at 55—normal). Her annual exam was delayed, as Angela's sister had come down with breast cancer, and she felt she needed to be with her. The sister lived some distance away, and alone. We discussed her continued estrogen use. She was now past the average age of menopause. She elected to continue estrogen, though she wanted to consult someone as well about a trial of tamoxifen. She was having some problems with tendonitis in the right shoulder and was referred for physical therapy. Her blood pressure now required a second drug. Her father, she reminded me, had had hypertension.

She continued with variable success to try to cut down on smoking. She tried an unsuccessful estrogen taper. Hot flashes were unbearable. We continued to weigh the risks together. Eventually, over a decade ago, her exam was normal—but this year, her mammogram was not. She needed excisional biopsy, which returned showing several foci of invasive lobular cancer and ductal carcinoma in situ (DCIS) in her right breast. She elected to have a mastectomy and immediate reconstruction. She had a favorable prognosis. She had to taper her hormones, and this was very difficult. Two months after her mammogram, and one month after her biopsy, she underwent mastectomy and immediate reconstruction with a tissue expander in place. The surgery went well, and pathology reports were quite favorable.

One month after her surgery, however, she came to the office in a high state of anxiety. Her surgical site had healed well, she did not need chemotherapy, and she had started her sessions with the plastic surgeon, a capable man who had much experience with breast reconstruction. Her tissue expander had to be gradually injected with increasing amounts of fluid to stretch and mold her healing mastectomy site for the future implant. The surgeon, she explained, stood behind her to inject the fluid. At the first session, she had taken her husband. Now, as she was a day away from her second visit, she was terrified, and couldn't understand it—embarrassed, but disabled. Why was this happening to her?

Was this process painful? Not unduly so. Did she trust the surgeon's experience and expertise? Absolutely. Was having her husband with her the right decision? Yes. Was the staff helpful? Very much so—very reassuring and comforting. Was she still in favor of reconstruction? Yes. So, Angela, I asked, was there not a history of sexual abuse in your background? An expression of shock and recognition. When she was eight years old, her father used to stand in front of her, expose his genitals, and masturbate. This happened repeatedly. When Angela's mother found out about it, she divorced him. As we know, this father had then pretty much disappeared from her life. Angela had thought she had "dealt with" this situation in her prior marital counseling and her own therapy. As we know, she had even courageously tried to converse with her father about it—from her point of view, unsuccessfully. Her reality was denied. Her general response to troubles was and is to "*put them behind*" her. Life was to be lived going forward. Things happen, you deal the best you can, then you put on a smile, personality, clothes—and go on, upbeat. The intimate relationship with this surgeon (whose reputation was impeccable, and who genuinely likes women) and the need for repeated "injections" had "blown her cover," so to speak—and she was paralyzed with fear.

I gave Angela a small amount of alprazolam to take, one before each procedure. Would she feel comfortable talking to the doctor about this? No. Should I? Absolutely not. How about his nurse? . . . yes. The nurse was a trusted older woman, somehow not unlike her own mother. (Angela did not always find her mother a source of reliable support, as we know. But her mother had, at a critical point, believed her daughter and removed her from harm's way.) It would be alright for me to call the surgeon's nurse and tell her what was going on, trusting her to keep the information to herself, and help Angela through the saline expansions.

Things weren't over for Angela, however. A month after we had worked on getting her through her treatments—and she was going now, with anxiety at a minimum—she was plagued by generalized anxiety and nightmares. The nightmares involved lying in her bed, hearing either her husband or her father climbing the stairs toward her bedroom. She experienced repeated terror. Nightmares were occurring with great regularity. In addition, she had developed some left lower quadrant pain and bowel disturbance, and on examination had a tender pelvic mass. CT scan demonstrated a small diverticular abscess—treatment of which would at the very least postpone the planned surgical reconstruction and was of some small concern regarding seeding of the expansion apparatus. In seeing her after the CT scan, she asked me to talk to the plastic surgeon not only about that—but about her abuse situation as well. Previously, she had not wanted him to know what was going on. It had been too embarrassing and as well, she did not want him to be distracted by his own feelings or concerns about him and her. Now—she needed him to know. She thought she might re-enter counseling as well.

A day or two later, I discussed Angela with the plastic surgeon. One reason that I admire and like this man is that he was comfortable with this information, not frightened of it. He seemed almost to welcome the challenge this situation provided to him. In turn, he had his own experience to share. "You know, taking care of these breast cancer patients is a tricky business," he reflected. Years ago, he spent months working with another breast reconstruction patient, a somewhat isolated professional woman. They were near the end of his treatment when she came in one day reporting that the oncologist had told her she was "done" with him for a year—she was doing well. "Well, this must be your lucky day!" he had replied. "You're done with me too!" This was a Friday, and he was on call for the weekend. The next day, he received a page from the medical examiner. "How often does that happen to a plastic surgeon?" he asked me. His patient had killed herself, leaving *his card* as the only medical information in her wallet. "Had this been expected?" queried the M.E. Not at all—but now, he said, he never severs a relationship with a reconstruction patient.

One can only wonder how his experience intertwined with Angela's. Here was a doctor bearing his own burden of pain, shock, and responsibility. Here was a patient whose "right side" and whose family history had been foreshadowing disease for years. Something about their collaboration freed Angela's story, and, as it turned out, the surgeon's, to be worked on a bit more out in the open between them.

Angela's gut did not yet require surgery. After reviewing her CT and discussing her situation with a trusted general surgeon, I treated her with antibiotics and diet. Nine days later, feeling better on antibiotics, the abscess ruptured through her vaginal cuff, leaving a healing drainage pathway from her peritoneum through her vagina. We elected to let her heal conservatively. She saw me three times following the completion of antibiotics to assess the drainage site and its healing. This required regular vaginal exams, which she tolerated with good humor. Ultimately, she did well. The plastic surgeon remained in touch, declaring himself "willing to wait as long as necessary." Three months after her first abdominal symptoms, she had uneventful reconstructive surgery.

I saw Angela a month after reconstruction. Somehow, in all of this, her nightmares and anxiety had diminished. She had planned to seek counseling but no longer felt the need to do so. However, ever the woman, she was "not happy" with her new breast. She worried a little about confronting the plastic surgeon about this, but she was "determined to get what she wanted." Her breast looked fine to her lying down, but not standing up. She wanted a re-do. On the other hand—she felt a bit washed out. Did I think she should do it? Should she wait? (And how to confront the surgeon? And was her anger okay?)

In due time, Angela respectfully made her request; the surgeon respectfully acknowledged the need for improvement, the re-reconstruction got done, patient and surgeon were satisfied, and the breast cancer, to date, has stayed away.

What can we learn from this case? What features of all our relationships with each other helped Angela navigate several serious threats—paralyzing anxiety, cancer, abdominal abscess, several surgeries—ultimately without permanent damage?

From my point of view, knowing that Angela was a trauma survivor was extremely helpful. That knowledge was there when the inscrutable but disabling anxiety showed up. Knowing, also, that trauma memories can literally burst into awareness, triggered by cues understandable only in retrospect, can help the provider act rightly in such an emergency. It is not unusual to have a trauma patient suddenly find him/herself flooded with negative feelings, needing emergent help to order them, act in a helpful way upon them, and proceed with what must be done. In addition, whatever help there is must be concordant with the *patient's* views on who is to be trusted and what should happen next. As Herman stresses, the patient must be in charge of her own recovery.

What seemed to help Angela? Her mother had rid the family of the father and ended the abuse, whatever other faults she might have had as a parent. The patient was able to build a trusting relationship which included some knowledge of herself as an abuse survivor. The patient had a clear sense of who (the surgeon's nurse) should know of the reasons for her anxiety. The surgeon had an above-average level of comfort in his role in working with a trauma patient. He could keep doing what he had to do, even though burdened with her information—her vulnerability, her projections, her experience of him as the "man climbing the stairs." His trauma with his prior patient was something he could readily bring to mind, perhaps as a way of understanding what sudden shock and dread feel like. Was his dead patient also an abuse survivor, who needed him more than either knew?

Angela "put things behind her"; this was how I coined her defensive style. Did her anxiety at having her surgeon also "behind her" stem from this? Whatever had happened, her ways of encasing her trauma had broken down; the present fused with the past. That this episode would bring into play all of her sexual organs—breast, genitals, brain, and mind—is nothing short of amazing. Her repeated dream evoked for her and me the helplessness and terror of her own abuse experience. In the dream, she is the little girl waiting for the inevitable perversion of her father. She is also herself, watching herself as an object of cruelty. In her life, she had freely chosen the route of reconstruction, which meant having her breast exposed repeatedly to others, just like her father exposed himself to her. She may not, at the outset, have thought that all the way through in making her decision to go for it. Ultimately, however, she used her anger healthily to get what she really wanted.

There are lessons here for all of us. They include: the importance of triggers; the need to let the patient set the agenda; the respect we must all have for the wisdom of the body, whose foreshadowing in this case passed all of our understanding; the need for curiosity and emotional resilience in dealing with the current realities reflecting past violence. We should note how we all had a role in her drama. We all created, and lived: the mother who knows and acts (rescuer); the mother who did not know soon enough (bystander); the abuser (who stood behind her in reality, but too much in front of her in the past); the abuser who would have to be faced repeatedly (the man climbing the stairs); the child/adult victim; the abuser as victim (of his patient, who killed herself when "abandoned"); the adult self who wants to forget it all, as we all must acknowledge would be easier; the terrified child; the brutalized child who wishes revenge ("I'm sorry, but that breast isn't good enough"). Such stories will and must be lived and enacted in our quest to care for each other.

References

1. Neruda P, "Poetry," in Housden R (ed.) *Risking Everything, 110 Poems of Love and Revelation*, pp. 8–9, Harmony Books, New York, 2003.
2. Alpert EJ, "Violence in intimate relationships and the practicing internist: new 'disease' or new agenda?," *Annals of Internal Medicine* 123(10): 774–781, 1995.
3. Alaggia R, "An ecological analysis of child sexual abuse disclosure: considerations for child and adolescent mental health," *Journal of the Canadian Academy of Child and Adolescent Psychiatry* 19(1): 32–39, 2010.
4. Bala M, "Caring for adult survivors of child sexual abuse: issues for family physicians," *Canadian Family Physician* 40: 925–931, 1994.
5. Davies M, Rogers P, "Perceptions of blame and credibility towards victims of childhood sexual abuse," *Journal of Child Sex Abuse* 18 (1): 78–92, 2009.
6. Herman J, *Trauma and Recovery*, p. 1, Basic Books, 1992.

7. Campling P, "Working with adult survivors of child sexual abuse," *British Medical Journal* 305: 1375–1376, 1992.
8. Plakun EM, "Enactment and the treatment of abuse survivors," *Harvard Review of Psychiatry* 5: 318–325, 1998.
9. Suchman AL, "A new theoretical foundation for relationship-centered care, complex responsive processes of relating," *Journal of General Internal Medicine* 21: 540–544, 2006.
10. Adler HM, "Toward a biopsychosocial understanding of the patient-physician relationship: an emerging dialogue," *Journal of General Internal Medicine* 22: 280–285, 2007.
11. Egnew TR, "Suffering, meaning, and healing: challenges of contemporary medicine," *Annals of Family Medicine* 7(2): 170–175, 2009.

9

Abuse, Violence, and Medical Care

Toward a Trauma-Informed System

> ***ER Doctor:*** *Have you ever been threatened or hurt by (. . .) or someone close to you?*
> ***Patient:*** *Yeah.*
> *(19-second pause)*
> ***ER Doctor:*** *Are you allergic to any medicine?* (1)

———

I want to be with people who submerge
in the task, who go into the fields to harvest
and work in a row and pass the bags along,
who stand in the line and haul in their places,
who are not parlor generals and field deserters
but move in a common rhythm
when the food must come in or the fire be put out.

The work of the world is common as mud.
Botched, it smears the hands, crumbles to dust.
But the thing worth doing well done
has a shape that satisfies, clean and evident.

Greek amphoras for wine or oil,
Hopi vases that held corn, are put in museums
but you know they were made to be used.
The pitcher cries for water to carry
and a person for work that is real. (2)

Introduction

Countless interactions among patients, providers, technology, treatments, and tools occur each day in our country. Provider–patient interactions, as discussed in Chapter 8, form a subset of these events. Outcomes of such relationships create one of the structures undergirding the system, conceived of as guiding it toward the best approximation of each "consumer's" health. How providers communicate (or not), how we function together, how we share our knowledge and lack of it, how we investigate and rectify our and our patients' problems, and how we structure and use our tools for caring for people form the nexus that I will call our health care system, for the purposes of this chapter.

Many say our system is "broken," and it may well be. It costs too much. Many people are still unable or unwilling to access it. Trying to provide affordable access to care has been the center of a giant political battle for over years. The system's end results are both spectacular, drawing patients from all over the world, and incredibly mediocre: our infant mortality rates in 2010 were higher than those of 26 other developed countries (3). We put solutions into place, such as Medicare or electronic health records, but then plunge into them while unintended and unforeseen consequences multiply around us. We spend years, billions of dollars, and much energy trying to rework what goes wrong. We leave solutions to the market and then feel powerless before the forces we have unleashed. We need leadership going forward, but as a country don't know whom, or whose vision, to trust.

In the face of such beauty and chaos, I will confess my own sense of smallness, but I put forth my contribution nonetheless. We need clear goals and a road map toward them. I would submit that our system and its practitioners need much more knowledge, skill, and systemic support for dealing with human trauma and its aftermath. There is evidence that our workforce lacks such knowledge, which must include self-knowledge. There are practices, sub-systems, and researchers who have begun to explore how to put such knowledge, if it is given, to work. We have some information on what the bumps in the road might be and how to deal with them. And we already have functioning examples of small systems in which such knowledge is bearing fruit. Some of them have been mentioned in previous chapters.

In reviewing what is known, I will broaden our scope to include all sorts of trauma—past and present. In searching the recent literature, I encountered next to nothing about creating a system that would support specifically adults with childhood histories of sexual violence. This may be appropriate, for several reasons. When thinking about a system to care for a population, we need to think about the needs of all peoples. It is true that the subset of people with childhood abuse has particular needs; but it is also true that trauma of all kinds engenders certain common dysfunctional responses in people—certain severe vulnerabilities, certain common suffering. We can expect to encounter patients with post-traumatic syndromes, high rates of addiction, various dissociative responses, and premature coronary disease, for example, among many populations, including our veterans, elders, survivors of motor-vehicle accidents, pro football players, children, witnesses and victims of domestic violence and neighborhood crime . . . the list goes on. I venture to guess, as well, that the subset of health care professionals includes many well-intentioned people with a history of various such traumas in various states of repair or disrepair.

Training

Wathen et al. (4) surveyed all college and university programs in Ontario, both undergraduate and postgraduate, which provided education to future health care professionals, asking whether they included training on intimate partner violence (IPV). She had a 95% response rate. Overall, 57% of programs provided any curriculum about IPV, not all of which were required. Significant barriers cited by leaders of these programs, not surprisingly, included funding and time. "Health care restructuring" was also cited as a barrier. Instructors who were knowledgeable, prepared, resourced, committed, AND who had time to update and renew their materials were cited as key to the presence and success of such curricula.

Significantly, nursing programs led the group in provision of instruction on partner violence. Twenty-five percent of postgraduate (residency) programs in medicine. and zero percent of such programs in dentistry, had such instruction. Less than half of the programs for doctors required attendance. Generally, across programs, from one to four hours were spent on the topic per year. Wathen concludes, among other things, "This suggests that physicians, one of the key types of health care professionals encouraged to intervene in cases of IPV, may not have sufficient educational opportunities in their primary training to become adequately knowledgeable, clinically competent, or comfortable in assessing and responding to IPV. . . . Although integrated, longitudinal, multi-disciplinary and experiential approaches to IPV education as advocated by experts in this area may be emerging in some programs, they are not yet evident, with one exception, in Ontario's post-secondary institutions."

Starling et al. (5) surveyed program directors and third-year residents at 67 US postgraduate training programs in family medicine, pediatrics, and emergency medicine regarding training programs, knowledge, and comfort of residents in managing childhood physical and sexual abuse. Surveying current knowledge, she cited the tendency for under-trained physicians to show "patterns of under-reporting, overreporting, and misdiagnosing maltreatment" of children. Over two-thirds of pediatric residents surveyed reported more than seven hours of clinical training, and experience with at least seven patients, with allegations of physical abuse, during their programs to date. Half of the residents had had experience with at least seven patients alleging sexual abuse. On the other hand, one-fifth or less of family medicine residents had the same exposure. Emergency residents reported similar low levels of clinical training as family medicine residents but had had middling exposure (41% and 33%) to at least seven patients in the categories above.

The survey included a 24-item quiz assessing residents' knowledge of child abuse evaluation. Future pediatricians did best. Family physicians did worst. Factors which improved resident performance included size of the program (larger was better); having a medical provider, center, interdisciplinary team, or faculty member focused on child abuse within the program; and requiring a rotation in child abuse. The setting of the program, and whether or not there was a university affiliation, seemed to make no difference. "Ultimately," she concludes, "residents should receive enough training to ensure that they can accurately identify and report abuse when it is suspected. Our study suggests that current levels of training are not meeting this critical goal. . . . [P]rograms that cannot provide adequate exposure to child abuse patients on site should establish clinical training opportunities at nearby child abuse programs or facilities with higher child abuse caseloads so that residents without the benefit of an on-site child abuse rotation can get at least minimal exposure to abused patients." Starling expresses hope that the ACGME will accredit a fellowship in child abuse pediatrics, which could lead to greater leadership and dissemination of knowledge among programs.

Family medicine programs fared better in a study of elder abuse education by Wagenaar et al. (6). She surveyed directors of 43 primary care residency programs (including family medicine, internal medicine, emergency medicine, and preventive medicine). Curriculum content and delivery methods, awareness of community resources, and "clinical contact" were examined, with a 63% response rate. Cluster analysis was performed based on amount of training and coverage of content. Internal medicine programs generally provided the least exposure; emergency medicine programs were somewhat higher, and family medicine trainees were said to have the highest level of training.

"Family medicine was characterized as having greater lecture topic variety, more clinical experiences in elder abuse, and greater use of screening tools for practice. Family medicine programs placed a higher degree of importance on the topic of elder abuse in their curriculum than did internal medicine residency programs. . . . Nearly all of the programs in the high-intensity group required elder abuse lecture attendance while none of the low-intensity groups required attendance. . . . The mean quality of training lectures was significantly different for clusters. . . . Lecture quality was rated on the basis of being practical, comprehensible, and retainable." Noting that "abused older patients often present in primary care offices, it is of concern that many primary care programs lack education in elder abuse presentation or care." Wagenaar also noted the lack, in clinical practice, of a reliable screening tool for elder abuse.

Finally, Nicolaidis et al. (7,8) have reported on a novel training program developed to improve health care workers' attitudes about and empathy for survivors of domestic violence. Noting that "physicians often waver between underestimating the impact of violence on their patients' lives and feeling overwhelmed by their inability to fix what appears to be a hopeless situation," she worked with experts in the field *and* victims, to create a documentary that would feature what survivors needed their doctors to know and feel. She then studied its impact in use in a group of recruited primary care practices in one county in Oregon.

Involving practices in the study was difficult. ". . . [I]nitial recruitment letters mailed to primary care providers and follow-up phone calls produced no response." Ultimately, a personal visit by a project member and follow-up phone calls produced a 34% response rate for this two-hour, free program. The program consisted of selected providers, support staff, and administration from each practice viewing the documentary and having a facilitated discussion, followed by a one-hour training on the clinical care of domestic violence patients. Despite the initial and ongoing reluctance, 96% rated the training as excellent to outstanding. Participant providers felt the training increased their sense of responsibility to screen, their confidence in doing so, their knowledge of what to do, and improved their assessment behavior. Affiliated staff and administrators also felt more responsible and knowledgeable, and staff gained empathy for clients undergoing domestic violence. Nicolaidis' view was that all staff members of a practice contribute to the culture of caring and concern.

Practice

Education is necessary and, it would seem, currently often deficient. Despite the lack, some practices and systems proceed. Gutmanis et al. (9), again working in Ontario, surveyed doctors and nurses about their knowledge and behavior when faced with a case scenario involving potential domestic violence. Roughly 33% of nurses and 42% of physicians said they initiated discussions about domestic violence routinely. Doctors were more likely to initiate discussions if they were emergency physicians (53%) than if they were in primary care specialties (25%).

Among doctors and nurses who had received training or education, three variables influenced how prepared the professional felt he was to bring up the issue: level of experience working with domestic abuse survivors; having a friend/relative/self involved in the issue, and having ever called the Children's Aid Society (presumably to report a current abuse situation). Gutmanis reported that "almost 50% of respondents indicated that they, a friend, or a relative had had experience with abuse, highlighting the prevalence of this issue." She also cited Feder (10), who in analyzing studies of women's experience disclosing to providers stated that such patients require that providers "have a full understanding of the issue of domestic violence, including knowledge of community services and appropriate referrals." Feeling prepared and **being** prepared are both important.

Roelens et al. (11) surveyed obstetricians in Belgium about knowledge and practice regarding domestic violence. Most greatly underestimated the prevalence of domestic violence among their populations and greatly overestimated their ability to detect it, relying on signs of physical abuse. As such, they were not in favor of universal screening (e.g., during pregnancy, during which there is an estimated risk of partner violence of 3%–4%). Despite this, they did endorse that such violence was not just a family affair, nor was it in their opinion the victim's fault. 50–60% felt unskilled and under-resourced were they to need to deal with a report of violence. Two-thirds of them felt they had not seen a case of it in the past five years. (The author estimated that the average practitioner in this survey would see a domestic violence patient once a month.)

Looking at a large set of variables—age, gender, time since board certification, volume of patients, hours worked/week, education/training, hospital type, and knowledge of a peer with an abuse history—only training was correlated with a self-report of asking every pregnant patient at least once during her prenatal care about domestic violence.

The authors admitted that education was necessary but insufficient at changing physician behaviors; they suggested "enabling tools" (screens) and reinforcement strategies, including feedback about providers' own behavior. In my experience, such strategies take time, persistence, and dedicated leadership. Per Roelens et al., "The crux of intimate partner violence is really that most women who encounter some kind of coercion will not present with overt signs of abuse, but rather with a wide variety of vague and nonspecific symptoms, if any." They also acknowledge a dearth of studies on the effectiveness (improved health and welfare) of any kind of screening for domestic violence but advocated for it nevertheless, citing expert opinion, the infectious nature of violence (effects for a lifetime on not just partners but children), the positive effect on care and the provider/client relationship of improved knowledge, and the low risk of harm in asking.

Bonds et al. (12) also noted the US Preventive Services Task Force (USPSTF) survey of the literature (13) as "insufficient to recommend screening" but cited a variance in opinions on the subject, including those from patients. Her group studied a multimodal intervention with a group of primary care practices in rural North Carolina. The goal was to increase reported screening for domestic violence. They were successful, increasing screening reported by patients from 16% of patient episodes to 26% of patient episodes, using tactics including training in-practice leaders, educating providers, reinforcing learning with regular teaching sessions during the study, paying the practice a stipend for participation, and customizing the intervention to the perceived needs of each practice's clientele.

Rhodes et al. (1) studied providers at two emergency department teams in Philadelphia which had an "enabling tool"—a computerized health risk assessment tool used on females ages 18–65 who were non-emergent and able to consent. The trial took place over six months, before which the 90 providers had 1.5 hours of updated instruction about assessing safety and providing referrals for domestic violence cases. The providers, mostly physician staff and physicians in training, knew that the goal was to increase detection of domestic violence. Visits were audiotaped; 293 of the 871 audiotapes contained a domestic violence discussion, and of these, 77 contained a disclosure (of which less than one-third had subsequent documentation of this disclosure in their chart).

Rhodes' group studied provider "communication strategies" which seemed to facilitate disclosure. They noted that a majority of discussions positive for domestic violence began because of a provider inquiry. "Patient disclosure of abuse was more likely to be found in audiotapes in which the provider probed for domestic violence, created open-ended opportunities for discussion, and was generally responsive or expressed empathy when a patient mentioned a psychosocial issue (for example, "stress"). Conversely, "meaningful conversations" in their opinion were limited by provider factors including "screening the patient in the presence of a third party, failure to acknowledge disclosure of abuse, lack of assessment of safety or level of risk, and failure to link the patient with available resources." Interrupting the patient, laughing, and use of professional wording all discouraged a discussion. Observing the awkwardness or "shutting-down" of some responses, they reiterated that "survivors report that validation of abuse, and encouragement by a health care provider can be life-changing if it is done without judgment—that is, when suggestions, not demands, are made."

Integrated Practice

There are many reasons why—at least back in 2004, the year of the USPSTF "recommendation"—there could be a lack of research demonstrating benefit from screening for the presence of violence in patients' lives. Liebschutz et al. (14) tackled some of these head on. She acknowledged the reality of negative consequences of health care encounters with professionals lacking adequate training. She also noted the tendency for research to focus on disclosure rather than improved quality of life. In a qualitative study of a small number of women survivors of partner abuse, she delved further into the impact of the patient–provider encounter on her subjects' lives.

Liebschutz and her group studied 25 subjects and 59 encounters with direct providers in the emergency room, ob-gyn, or primary care offices. The patients themselves labeled consequences of disclosure as beneficial, harmful, or unhelpful; researchers categorized the encounters as disclosures, discovery (provider knew, and patient knew that provider knew), and non-disclosures. There were no disclosures that resulted in "actual" harm to patients; however, participants on nine occasions reported that disclosure was unhelpful, generating fear for their lives, a severance of ongoing relationship with a provider, and avoidance of health care, as well as a perception that providers were uninvolved or uninformed.

In contrast, 44% of beneficial enclosures led directly to a change in the participant's circumstances, such as leaving the abusive spouse, entering a detoxification program, or filing a police report. For example, one participant with newborn twins and a toddler reported that after disclosing her husband's assaults, "I started off in a shelter in (a distant town) because I couldn't find one that would take all of us right away. . . . My (OB) got on the phone with Social Service to try and get me all the help that I needed."

Others resulted in "a shift in the participant's self-esteem, perception of the violent relationship, or awareness of alternatives, eventually empowering her to seek help for the abuse on her own." Notably, these study participants were recruited from IPV survivor programs, so that the number of "beneficial" encounters may be elevated compared to an average patient population.

Notably, disclosures were much more likely to be beneficial in provider relationships that involved long-term care (such as ob-gyn and primary care) as opposed to emergency department encounters. Liebschutz postulated that comfort, trust, and mutual respect were the basis of progress in the former. Those factors can be developed in the emergency room as well, and sometimes were. However, patients in emergency departments are more likely to be frightened, in pain, and vulnerable; in addition, the nature of emergency work precludes sustained attention to one individual's problems, save for a life-threatening situation.

Interestingly, Liebschutz investigated the benefits and harms of situations where abused women presented for care but did not disclose. A common thread here was the importance of a perception (by patients) that caregivers knew that violence had occurred, were familiar with the concept of domestic violence, and/or demonstrated care about the patient's welfare. The presence of these factors enabled some women to take action for themselves at a later time, when they felt ready. In contrast, their absence generated a belief that the doctor did not care, and sometimes a severance of the relationship, with no progress on ending the violence in the woman's life.

In primary care settings, clinicians and researchers report barriers to achieving the kinds of outcomes in their trauma patients that Liebschutz describes. Gerber et al. (15), working in two public hospital clinic settings, found that 18% of primary clinicians did not consider it their job to screen for intimate partner violence. Of the great majority who did, however, many reported a lack of confidence in handling such cases, despite having confidence in their skills in other physical and psychological domains. Even when presented with a written, positive domestic violence screen administered in their waiting room that same day, 28% of clinicians failed to note any evidence of the screen in their subsequent note, and only 10% detailed what had happened to the patient and documented a safety plan.

In several studies of providers, confidence in handling issues involving violence rose, not surprisingly, proportionate to the practitioner's volume of such cases and to his or her training. We have to admit to ourselves that the first step in arriving at such skill and experience is to acknowledge the presence of present and past violence in the lives of our patients, whatever our self-perceived shortcomings are.

Practicing within a network of informed co-workers is also important. In an interesting Dutch study about handling trauma in general in their patients, van den Akker et al. (16) found that GPs reported increasing difficulty depending on the type of trauma: 63% felt few barriers in helping patients who had survived physical accidents, whereas 52% felt confident facing domestic violence victims and only 40% with cases involving current child abuse. In all cases where barriers were experienced, the general practitioners felt they lacked a relationship with or awareness of specialists with more expertise in the area. They wanted, as well, improved training for themselves in handling such things as suspecting and detecting abuse, raising the subject with their patients, and confronting parents.

Training, experience, and support are most certainly important, as is overcoming the perception that violence has not or is not occurring in patients' lives. However, there are some fundamental principles within the grasp of most of us that exist and have been laid out. Battaglia et al. (17), studying "safe and productive" disclosure of partner abuse in the health care setting, emphasized the following provider characteristics as beneficial: the ability to communicate concern, willingness to negotiate control, assurance of confidentiality, medical competence, careful listening, and taking enough time. Many of these are integral to our identity as physicians, and others are at least somewhat under our control. Monahan and Forgash (18), teaching about caring for the population of adult female survivors of child sexual abuse, remind us about the importance of understanding the patient's point of view around issues of touch (may be experienced as "invasive, intrusive and noxious"); low self-esteem (patient feeling unworthy of help, or living in an environment where the harm was confusingly denied); power and control (see Chapter 5); triggering and re-experiencing during medical procedures; and very high and very low pain thresholds.

Finally, Mollica (19), writing of the growing population of refugees in our nation, points out the salience of trauma in the lives of such people. "It is our experience working with traumatized patients that the traumatic life events of the patient must be a central focus of clinical thinking. . . . Demonstrating to patients that their trauma story is an important component of their medical history is a significant step in establishing rapport." He advocates putting the "trauma history" at the top of the problem list because of its ability to infuse all other aspects of a patient's life, especially when losses—of physical integrity, of family members including children, of professional and social standing—are involved.

Personal Issues for Health Care Providers

It should be clear by now that trauma of all sorts afflicts us all with a sense of loss. The losses to victims have been enumerated. But health care providers are also among the bereaved. In the studies above, at least, doctors working with the traumatized seem to experience a loss of perceived competence, in some cases a loss of compassion for self and others, and a loss of a sense of a competent community of practitioners. I think this mirrors our patients' experiences of trauma, which robs people of physical and mental integrity, self-worth, and identification with their families and communities, among other things.

Pross (20) has written of such "vicarious traumatization" in health care. He suggests that unguarded work with trauma patients can lead to "burnout," characterized by "apathy, feelings of hopelessness, rapid exhaustion, disillusionment, melancholy, forgetfulness, irritability, experiencing work as a heavy burden, alienated, impersonal, uncaring and cynical attitude towards clients, tendency to blame oneself, and feeling(s) of failure." He discusses "professional cynicism," which helps people in all fields confronted with the day-to-day stresses of their jobs but which, when magnified, "turns into brutalization and contempt" and is a hallmark of health care relationships in which the provider has succumbed to the trauma of his job.

Pross quotes Hoppe (21), who studied those who evaluated the post-release experiences of concentration camp victims in the 1950s and 1960s. Hoppe noted that the (German) evaluators evolved four defensive styles in dealing with the stories they heard. These included denial, rationalization, over-identification, and "controlled identification." Hoppe felt the last was ideal, because it resulted in fair assessments and effective reparations for the victim in the society at large. Deniers minimized the victims' current sufferings in order to deal with their own fear and guilt at the stories they heard. Rationalizers appeared pleasant to the victims, and in so doing assuaged their own shame, but then wrote "objective, scientific" reports failing to find links between camp experiences and current disabilities. Over-identifiers linked themselves with the victims, magnified and polemicized their reports, and virtually guaranteed failure of compensation by lack of objectivity. Rather than aiding victims they were expressing their own hatred of the oppressors, and disappointment in themselves for not overcoming their own failures in relationship to them. Controlled identifiers withheld judgment, believed the victims' stories no matter how incredible, allowed themselves to feel the terror that their victims felt, but also "observe(d) (themselves) critically." I think that last point is crucial—the ideal evaluators reserved critical evaluation for themselves—not for the victims.

Pross also cites studies linking personality and motivations of providers to burnout. People may enter the health care professions not just altruistically but also to seek power (and avoid feelings of powerlessness), to work and help to excess (and avoid one's own neediness), to avoid fears of illness and death, to seek glory and honor (and avoid contempt of oneself), and finally, to control people with violent and destructive activities (and control one's own violent tendencies and overwhelming despair). If in the course of training and self-knowledge, these impulses and needs are not recognized and channeled, they will appear in the course of work, over-expressed, and lead to exhaustion, self-recrimination, isolation, or malfeasance.

Finally, Pross notes that those who work with trauma victims often suffer from a "low level of social recognition, especially in the professional establishment." On the one hand this can lead to the setting up of special centers and clinics to deal with trauma victims, which can undergird a sense of excitement and specialness on the part of providers. On the other hand, when no one is listening, when promotions and recognition are denied, and when pay is low, this by itself can lead to burnout. He strongly recommends integration of trauma treatment into every day of professional life for these reasons.

Domestic violence affects women more than men. Those who write for us about its treatment are often women. Wong et al. (22), a mixed-gender group, reported on the effects of provider gender on responding to partner abuse. They studied Dutch family practitioners using single-sex focus groups with a same-sex moderator, a "senior social scientist . . . with no special interest in domestic violence." Eight questions aimed at understanding provider attitudes were posed to six groups in all, including questions about practitioners' reactions to abuse, conceptualization of violence, and clinical experiences. Both male and female doctors believed that male dominance, accentuated in some cultural groups, and perpetrator's backgrounds of neglect and abuse, as well as substance abuse played a role in domestic violence. Doctors of both sexes often experienced powerlessness when faced with the issue and also feared aggression from the perpetrator when deciding whether to deal with it. They also felt conflicted when, as often, they were charged with providing care both to alleged victim and perpetrator.

There were also major differences between providers of the two sexes. Male doctors' groups endorsed beliefs that female victims played a role in violence by refusing sex, and evidenced conflict about the rights of women to limit male sexual advances. The female doctors were unanimous in their understanding of both the danger a woman may face in opposing a mate's sexual advances and the humiliation involved in coerced sexual relations. The men noted the repetitive behaviors of female victims (repeatedly choosing abusive partners); women felt leaving such relationships was a process, and repetition was not equated with failure. Men tended to deny difficulty discussing abuse with patients yet avoided emotional involvement with them; women doctors tended to have difficulties distancing themselves from patient's experiences and to feel overwhelmed if they were handling too many cases. Men felt they hardly ever saw any such cases; women reported their experiences in graphic detail. Women discussed and exchanged strategies for responding to patients; men were inclined to "theorize on how to respond." Reading this study, as a woman, I marveled at the limits of the professionalization process in affecting people of both genders' views about and skills at responding to violence in human relationships. The case below might explicate such limits.

Olivia

Olivia was an ICU nurse in her early 40s, married, without children, who loved her job and planned to make critical care her career. She gained experience and standing through the years and served on numerous patient care committees alongside other nurse and physician colleagues. She was dedicated to her job, often working after her shift to do her best to care for her patients and their families and to help her fellow nurses in times of crisis on the unit.

At home things were not as rosy. She had married in her early 30s to a man who was a research scientist. He was a little older than she, had more regular hours, and had the experience of being at home waiting for her, at which he often chafed. He wanted and needed more of her attention.

During much of her 20s, Olivia had experienced severe depression, even as she found her chosen career. Eventually she sought psychotherapy with a psychiatrist, twice a week, which stretched on for a number of years. Without her realizing what was happening, this man had become gradually and then regularly physically intimate with her, in the name of treating her fears of sexual function and human closeness. Olivia had felt very dependent on his attention and his opinions. She was devastated when he retired.

She met her future husband shortly after her therapist's retirement. Initially, love and passion helped her through the early stages of the sexual relationship. Gradually, however, she became less and less interested in sex. She and her husband were fighting about it and feeling more isolated from each other. She did not know why she felt this way, nor what to do.

Meanwhile, a few years after her therapy came to an end, this psychiatrist's behavior arrived on the front pages of the local newspaper. A lawsuit against her psychiatrist had been brought by another former client, who alleged that they had had sexual intercourse at his behest on a number of occasions. Olivia read the articles. With a shock, she realized that the therapy relationship had perhaps not been what she thought. She felt numb but knew that this was important. She wondered what, if anything, it had to do with her and her husband's problems.

Olivia consulted her primary care doctor about this question. Her doctor, who knew some of what trouble the couple was having and had wondered about prior abuse, knew of an ongoing therapy group comprising specifically patients previously abused by mental health professionals. It was local, ongoing, and expensive. Olivia wondered if her health insurance could pay. With her doctor's blessing, she decided to consult one of the male physicians she'd worked with over the years, who oversaw many aspects of the hospital's health insurance plan.

It was hard for Olivia to talk to this man. There was a great deal of mutual respect between them, having shared patients and committee tasks over the years. She had to run through her past treatment, which now had begun to feel shameful to her, and at least refer to her current marital issues. But she felt the group could be helpful. When she was done, there was a silence as this doctor looked at her. "Well, Olivia," he said, "I wish you hadn't told me." She did not know what to say.

Olivia brought this encounter back to her primary care doctor. Together, the two women wondered what this could mean. Did this man think he would no longer be able to respect Olivia? Was he implying that knowing what he did now, he could no longer be impartial? Was he saying that she, like other professionals, should know that this was not a topic for educated professionals to discuss? Was what had happened to her something he preferred to have her keep to herself, as opposed to being a wake-up call for the whole profession? Did he think it was her fault? Was he just trying to be humorous? Olivia doubted it.

Ultimately, he and the health plan agreed to cover the sessions. Olivia was relieved and went on to join the group. She reported to her primary care doctor that it was helpful. But she felt that professionally, this influential man thought that *she* had violated professional boundaries, and that she was now some sort of damaged object in his eyes. She knew that among her nurse colleagues, there were others who held trauma stories. She wondered whom she could trust. She wondered how this doctor had treated his own trauma patients, and what her hospital system felt about her and others like her.

I offer Olivia's example not to single out male professional behavior. I have heard this attitude—that prior abuse is nuisance information, degrading to its victim and to a professional relationship, or somehow at least irrelevant—from women health care providers as well. What I mean to do instead is to lift the curtain, for the health care system as a whole, on the denial and minimization we still live with as a profession and a society when it comes to human violence.

Other Provider Issues

A different type of difficulty for health service professionals is noted by Ryan et al. (23) writing of the co-opting of the profession by abusive birth and foster parents caring for developmentally disabled children. They wrote of the experiences of a Colorado consult team (developmental physician, psychiatrist, and behavior specialist) traveling to birth and foster care homes to consult with families and treating physicians caring for such children. Most families were doing the best they could. There were examples, however, of children locked in cages, restrained, bruised, starved, and sexually abused, in which their experienced and caring physicians had, at the behest of the parent, signed off on the treatment, effectively dooming the child to more abuse. These treating physicians had been lied to by parents; they found it hard to trust their gut feelings and observations generating suspicion; they relied on consultants' opinions rather than their own; they were threatened by social service agencies that contrary findings would threaten children's placement or "well-being"; and they were lulled into complacency by acceptance of treatment by (terribly overworked) social service agencies. The authors recommended ongoing training for physicians working in this area: not accepting decline in children's function as expected, home visits, time evaluating the child alone, and understanding the system of power in which they worked (who they could report to and get information from), among others. They cited Lifton's important work studying physicians' cooperating with and co-opting during the Nazi genocide, 1939–1945, which targeted Jews and developmentally disabled individuals with lives "not expected to contribute to the Aryan regime."

A possible consequence of practicing with abuse in mind was cited by Jenny (24), writing of the "intimidation of British pediatricians." She wrote of contemporary cases in which the British licensing board had threatened or removed the licenses of well-known child abuse pediatricians, and many more in which parents and others had filed formal complaints about child abuse pediatricians with the board, as a result of pediatricians' raising questions about child maltreatment. She cited numerous press attacks on, for instance, the validity of shaken baby syndrome. In the United States, respected professionals have raised the same questions. The matter is far from closed. Yet, both parents and pediatricians are tasked with protecting children from harm. If a health care professional has substantive concern, how is he to raise it? Jenny noted that in her setting, after a complaint, physicians were "hounded and insulted by the press," and she gave examples of coverage slanted heavily toward alleged abusers/parents. Jenny called for better education of the public and the press about the "realities of the diagnosis of child maltreatment."

In the United States, all states have laws mandating reporting of suspected child abuse—laws which govern behavior not just of health care providers but also school personnel, church personnel, and others. Such laws provide immunity from prosecution if such reports are made in good faith. What the law cannot provide is immunity from notoriety, wrath, and public misinformation programs. Parents and caretakers have legitimate rights and needs to protect themselves and their reputations. But abusers have a powerful interest in protecting their access to children; abusers often have large and important reputations to protect as well. Uncovering the lid on child abuse exposes the mandated reporter to the same tactics that victims have experienced at the hands of the abusers. True abusers are often persistent, believe in themselves, have many friends and supporters, and have many tactics to protect their behavior. Excellent training, sticking to one's job, reporting one's own observations and experiences are the tools the medical profession has in the face of this behavior. Truth is a powerful weapon but must be accompanied by training and a strong constitution. In addition, a provider should **never** be doing this kind of work alone.

Trauma-Informed Systems of Care

The study of disease and organ systems, the advent of the problem-oriented medical record, and the increased depth and specialization of medical and psychological knowledge during the 20th and 21st centuries have all led to incredible advances in our care of individuals, as well as major fragmentation and dysfunction in our systems of care. Every busy clinician knows the burden caused by a patient whose problems span organ systems, or whose behavior or beliefs preclude simple categorization and procedures. Specialization allows providers to avoid some of that burden, which then falls on generalists. Primary care practice is endangered when trainees and practitioners see it as a dumping ground at worst, or a triage system at best. This can cause interest in it to wither, as has happened since 1990.

Let's consider, then, how we might reinvigorate the practice and relieve some of the burden of those who care for the many complex patients whose lives have been corrupted by violence. We have seen how frequent they are in our waiting rooms, whether we acknowledge it or not. We have also touched on the tendency to marginalize such providers. It may be no coincidence that generalists, providing care for the many with inexplicable histories, vague complaints, and "psychosomatic" conditions, have also suffered from lower wages and recognition in the eyes of the profession.

This is going to require some creative "out of the box" thinking. Some interesting results have emerged from the Substance Abuse and Mental Health Services Administration, which in 1998 began the Women, Co-occurring Disorders and Violence Study (WCDVS). WCDVS looked at the effect of integrating treatment for substance abuse and mental health issues in women with histories of physical and sexual abuse. To participate in and receive funding for their studies, individual centers had to show that they could *integrate care* at the service level (care had to be simultaneous and coordinated). They also were required to provide services that *addressed the impact of trauma* in women's lives and *involve consumers* as facilitators of and consultants to the program. Finally, they were required to be *comprehensive*, providing such services as screening, parenting skills, peer counseling, and crisis intervention.

Many studies emerged from the WCDVS. In general, Morrissey et al. (25) revealed during this study that service integration (not just provision, but real integration) produced better health outcomes, particularly for drug addiction, measures of PTSD, and measures of mental health symptoms. Change was slow but measurable across a 12-month period. General medical care was not included in the treatment model and, not surprisingly, according to Chung et al. (26) clients evidenced no change in their interactions with hospitals and health care providers in terms of how often trauma, substance abuse, or mental health issues came up or were treated during the study. Noether et al. (27), writing about the study as a whole, raised many questions about how the participants changed, what order was followed, whether substance abuse always had to be addressed first, and how recovery in one domain influenced and affected other domains.

Mammen (28) writes of a process initiated by the Department of Psychiatry at St. Vincent's Hospital in Melbourne, Australia, a general teaching hospital. They were responding to a large increase in referrals of adults for treatment of symptoms related to childhood sexual abuse, and a perceived dearth of services for them. They organized several meetings of representatives of local health and welfare agencies, which resulted in the creation of a "sexual abuse resource group." This group met monthly for an educational and networking session for two years. They organized four training workshops for specific types of providers during the same time. They targeted community health centers, substance abuse workers, medical practitioners, and people who worked with youth for the training workshops. Mammen noted, "Medical practitioners appeared less aware of the relevance of childhood sexual abuse to emotional and physical problems, often considering it not relevant to the socioeconomic class of their particular clientele. Exceptions were women practitioners or others with a special interest. Males interested in working in the area often described a particular helplessness in dealing with issues of sexual abuse, particularly those involving women." She cited inadequate and variable training and lack of networking as deficits leading to poorly trained medical practitioners—factors they were attempting to remedy.

Gibbons (29), also writing from Australia, comments on the difficulties survivors of childhood abuse encounter trying to find satisfactory mental health counseling, citing studies that many consulted up to nine providers and that nearly two-thirds of the providers, when child sexual abuse was mentioned by the client, "didn't delve further." She noted declining funding for health and welfare services at the time, as well as difficulties survivors had in accessing the expertise that was present in the system. She cited studies showing 10%–23% of victims reporting subsequent sexual abuse by counselors they consulted for their sexual abuse issues. She advocated for a cost-neutral "reorientation of service provision." This would include agency acknowledgment of the frequency of abuse, supervision by experienced childhood sexual assault experts, and good management practices. She further stressed the importance of a supportive, valuing work environment in which the treating professionals are not abused by the agency or system itself.

Gibbons cited Armsworth, underlining practices professionals can enhance in themselves to be of help to women who have experienced domestic and sexual violence. Armsworth (30) outlined fundamentals of good care to victims:

1. The client (is) believed.
2. The professional (demonstrates) concern, care, empathy, compassion.
3. The client (is) not blamed for the victimization.
4. The professional (is) not shocked or disgusted at the incest disclosure.
5. The client (does) not feel alone or odd.
6. Where applicable, the professional helps to get the incest stopped.

Returning to the topic of male helplessness in the face of evidence of victimization of women, Gibbons suggests that "men in the helping professions could offer leadership in designing social action and preventive programmes to address male violence." Citing Russell, who stated that "sexual abuse of children, rape of females, and sexual harassment would be rare if males were socialized to be uninterested in having sexual contact with unwilling partners," she emphasizes that stopping sexual abuse involves more than children and women learning to say no. In our societies, men hold and hold on to real power over women, but it need not continue this way. Men, however, are needed to be part of stopping this.

Both men and women in the helping professions could further their care of victims by stopping the abuse of each other within the profession. Many professional communities are undermined by misuse of power and information. Often those who are interested in leadership are those least suited to creating communities that enhance excellence in each individual and promote dialogue as equals. Often it seems that our leaders are those who are blindly re-enacting some personal trauma of their own, immutable to insight and change. Men and women professionals each individually have a role in furthering self-awareness and promoting healthy conflict around this issue.

Chen et al. (31) reported on the efforts of one child protection team (CPT) within Safra Children's Hospital in Israel. Each hospital is mandated by the Israeli government to have such a team. Safra's was composed of one social worker, one pediatrician, a psychiatrist, and a nurse. In the course of their work, it became clear to them that the observations and knowledge of all the staff caring for the child were critical in understanding the child's true situation; yet the staff was under-trained, varied in their experience with abuse issues, and overworked. In response, they developed a weekly "roundtable" session, case-based, inviting *all* hospital workers and trainees to attend. "The discussion that ensues," the authors noted, "is an open and honest exchange, whereby the CPT seriously considers the staff's feedback. In addition to the educational and clinical aspects, given the ambiguous nature of many cases, the discussions serve the CPT itself as an informal auditing mechanism." Attendees developed improved knowledge and skills around the topic, greater understanding of policies, and improved sense of personal safety around reporting and acting on such cases.

Another example is that of Wain and Gabriel (32), who reported on the creation of a Preventive Medical Psychiatry Service (PMPS) at Walter Reed in the context of wars in Iraq and Afghanistan, nested within the psychiatry liaison services already existing. The task of the PMPS is to round with the medical and surgical team on every trauma patient, screening each one for psychiatric comorbidities and making routine for the patient and the treatment team the concept of doing so. Their strategies included normalizing the inevitable stress responses that soldiers develop, creating a therapeutic alliance, focusing on current hopes and realities, and attending to the importance of transference and counter-transference issues, partly to educate the non-psychiatric clinicians about patient–clinician interactions. For instance, one psychiatrist facing deployment initially avoided discussion of genital functioning with a soldier whose testicles had been destroyed by a bullet wound; he realized his own fears in supervision by the PMPS. The group educated the staff about personality traits and defense mechanisms, their place in the mental health of the patient, and how to understand and use these to further the patient's health (rather than object to, oppose, or pathologize them).

Finally, we can take note of the good work occurring in subsets of another large system of social care, our public schools. The states of Massachusetts and Washington have studied and published excellent manuals (33,34) on creating trauma-informed schools in response to the increases in numbers of students who are refugees, victims/witnesses of domestic violence, members of violent or impoverished communities, homeless, and more. Not surprisingly these students have trouble learning, as well as many behavioral and emotional problems which make standard approaches to education less effective. School personnel studied and made use of Felitti and Anda's work on Adverse Childhood Experiences, and Judith Herman's work on trauma and repair. They began to recognize that much of what they were seeing in their students had to do with fear, lack of trust, damaged brain circuitry, and lack of well-trained adult allies.

Administrators, principals, and teachers in alternative schools got together in these states, educated themselves, and began initiating, with remarkable success, approaches to education of traumatized youth of all ages. The state of Washington's manual identifies six principles of teacher and school behavior toward these young people:

1) Seek to empower, and avoid disempowerment.
2) Unconditional positive regard of the student (of his being, not necessarily of his actions).
3) Hold high expectations.
4) Examine your own assumptions, continue to observe and question.
5) Become a "relational coach."
6) Offer (students) guided opportunities to be helpful to others.

Principle 1 undergirds what has been presented in Chapter 5 on power. Principle 2 is implicit in what I've emphasized in a number of chapters but perhaps deserves special recognition. This concept, first enunciated by Carl Rogers, holds not just that this person is doing the best she can, but perhaps has its roots in the ideal beginning of life, as parents hold and regard their newborn child—a product of their positive joint effort, a miracle of creation, and the living representation of the work to be done to create the best human being possible. Principle 4 steers us toward self-questioning and continued thoughtful reflection. Principle 6 reminds us of the usefulness of the recovering victim to us as providers, to others in recovery, and to himself as he begins to give back.

This manual also devotes a chapter to the school–community partnership, which our health care system would be wise to emulate. It stresses the importance of engaging leadership at all levels, understanding and encouraging many systems to give and cooperate, offering training, continually reviewing and revising policies, and creating viable working relationships within various communities.

Central to all these efforts are several key components. Someone(s) in the system recognized that trauma had occurred and was rife in the lives of their clients. Leaders understood that clients were presenting problems to them and hoping for assistance, not just wreaking havoc. The teams involved eventually understood that the problems were theirs to solve. They convened and mobilized themselves across disciplines. They provided leadership and experimented with programs. Finally, they attempted to educate all relevant co-workers about what was learned—what worked, what did not, and why. They furthered knowledge and enriched the lives not only of the clients but of their co-workers. All of us can learn from their pioneering efforts. They have made not only their students' and schools' lives better, but by providing positive educational homes and building more resilient and competent students, they are contributing to a healthier society for us and our own children. They are part of healing trauma.

To do the best job for our traumatized patients, we need ongoing education and re-education. We need exposure to effective systems and leaders in the field. We need experiential learning to mold our behavior and systems. We need colleagues and ongoing mutual relationships with interested professionals inside and outside of health care. We in general medicine need time and recognition of the experience we have, and time to create the systems we need. We need to take the best care we can of ourselves and each other. We need to live our professional lives fully aware of the potential for human cruelty to destroy, and of our own potential to heal. We can only begin to realize that potential if we know what we are facing. And we will only really know what we are facing if we talk about it, and work on it, together.

References

1. Rhodes KV, Frankel RM, Levinthal N, Prenoveau E, Bailey J, and Levinson W, " 'You're not a victim of domestic violence, are you?' Provider-patient communication about domestic violence," *Annals of Internal Medicine* 147(9): 620–627, 2007.
2. "To be of use" from CIRCLES ON THE WATER by Marge Piercy, copyright © 1982 by Middlemarsh, Inc. Used by permission of Alfred A. Knopf, an imprint of the Knopf Doubleday Publishing Group, a division of Penguin Random House LLC. All rights reserved, 1982.
3. MacDorma MF, Mathews TJ, Mohangoo AD, and Zeitlin JZ, "International comparisons of infant mortality and related factors, US and Europe, 2010," *National Vital Statistics Reports* 63(5): 1–27, 2014.

4. Wathen CN, Tanaka M, Catallo C, Lebner AC, Friedman MK, Hanson MD, et al.; and, the McMaster IPV Education Research Team, "Are clinicians being prepared to care for abused women? A survey of health professional education in Ontario, Canada, *BMC Medical Education* 9: 1–15, 2009.
5. Starling S, Heisler KW, Paulson JF, and Youmann E, "child abuse training and knowledge: a national survey of emergency medicine, family medicine, and pediatric residents and program directors," *Pediatrics* 123(4): e595–e602, 2009.
6. Wagenaar DB, Rosenbaum R, Herman S, and Page C, "Elder Abuse Education in Primary Care Residency Programs: A Cluster Group Analysis," *Family Medicine* 41(7): 481–486, 2009.
7. Nicolaidis C, "The *Voices of Survivors* documentary, using patient narrative to educate physicians about domestic violence," *Journal of General Internal Medicine* 17: 117–124, 2002.
8. Nicolaidis C, Curry MA, and Gerrity M, "Measuring the impact of the *Voices of Surivivors* program on health care workers' attitudes toward survivors of intimate partner violence," *Journal of General Internal Medicine* 20(8): 731–737, 2005.
9. Gutmanis I, Beynon C, Tutty L, Wathen CN, and MacMillan HL, "Factors influencing identification of and response to intimate partner violence: a survey of physicians and nurses," *BMC Public Health* 7: Article 12, 2007.
10. Feder GS, Hutson N, Ramsay J, and Taket AR, "Women exposed to intimate partner violence: expectations and experiences when they encounter health care professionals; a meta-analysis of qualitative studies," *Archives of Internal Medicine* 166: 22–37, 2006.
11. Roelens I, Verstraelen H, Van Egmond K, and Temmerman M, "A knowledge, attitudes, and practice survey among obstetrician-gynecologists on intimate partner violence in Flanders, Belgium," *BMC Public Health* 6(238): 1–10, 2006.
12. Bonds DE, Ellis SD, Weeks E, Palla SL, and Lichstein P, "A practice-centered intervention to increase screening for domestic violence in primary care practices," *BMC Family Practice* 7(63): 1–10, 2006.
13. US Preventive Service Task Force, "Screening for family and intimate partner violence: recommendation statement," *Annals of Internal Medicine* 140: 382–386, 2004.
14. Liebschutz J, Battaglia T, Finley E, and Averbuch T, "Disclosing intimate partner violence to health care clinicians–what a difference the setting makes: A qualitative study," *BMC Public Health* 8(229): 1–11, 2008.
15. Gerber MR, Leiter KS, Hermann RC, and Bor DH, "How and why community hospital clinicians document a positive screen for intimate partner violence: a cross-sectional study," *BMC Family Practice* 6(48): 1–9, 2005.
16. van den Akker M, Mol S, Metsemakers J, Dinant G, and Knottnerus J, "Barriers in the care of patients who have experienced a traumatic event: the perspective of general practice, *Family Practice* 18: 214–216, 2001.
17. Battaglia T, Finley E, and Liebschutz JM, "Survivors of intimate partner violence speak out: trust in the patient-provider relationship," presented at SGIM 24th annual meeting, San Diego, CA, May 2001.
18. Monahan K and Forgash C, "Enhancing the health care experiences of adult female survivors of childhood sexual abuse," *Women and Health* 30(4): 27–41, 2000.
19. Mollica RF, "Surviving torture," *New England Journal of Medicine* 351(1): 5–7, 2004.
20. Pross C, "Burnout, vicarious traumatization and its prevention," *Torture* 16(1): 1–9, 2006.
21. Hoppe KD, "The emotional reactions of psychiatrists when confronting holocaust survivors of persecution," in: Lindon J (ed.) *Psychoanalytic Forum* III, p. 187. New York: Science House, 1969.

22. LoFong Wong, SH, DeJonge A, Wester F, Mol SS, Romkens RR, and Lagro-Janssen T, "Discussing partner abuse: does doctor's gender really matter?," *Family Practice* 23(5): 578–586, 2006.
23. Ryan R, Salbenblatt J, Schiappacasse J, and Maly B, "Physician unwitting participation in abuse and neglect of persons with developmental disabilities," *Community Mental Health Journal* 37(6): 499–509, 2001.
24. Jenny C, "The intimidation of British pediatricians," *Pediatrics* 119(4): 797–799, 2007.
25. Morrissey JP, Jackson EW, Ellis AR, Amaro H, Brown VB, and Najavits L, "Twelve-month outcomes of trauma-informed interventions for women with co-occurring disorders," *Psychiatric Services*; 56: 1213–1222, 2005.
26. Chung S, Domino ME, and Morrissey JP, "Changes in treatment content of services during trauma-informed integrated services for woman with co-occurring disorders," *Community Mental Health Journal* 45: 375–384, 2009.
27. Noether CD, Finkelstein N, VanDeMark NR, Savage A, Reed BG, and Moses DJ, "Design strengths and issues of SAMHSA's Women, Co-occurring Disorders, and Violence Study," *Psychiatric Services* 56(10): 1233–1236, 2005.
28. Mammen G, "Primary health care for adult survivors of childhood sexual abuse," *Australian and New Zealand Journal of Public Health*; 20(6): 649–653, 1996.
29. Gibbons J, "Services for adults who have experienced child sexual assault: improving agency response," *Social Science Medicine* 43(12): 1755–1763, 1996.
30. Armsworth MW, "Therapy of incest survivors: abuse or support?" *Child Abuse and Neglect* 13: 549, 1989.
31. Chen W, Bernout E, Tzur S, and Glasser S, "Roundtable sessions of a children's hospital child protection team," *Psychiatric Services* 59(693): 1–3, 2008.
32. Wain HJ and Gabriel GM, "Psychodynamic concepts inherent in a biopsychosocial model of care of traumatic injuries," *Journal of the American Academy of Psychoanalysis and Dynamic Psychiatry* 35(4): 555–573, 2007.
33. Cole SF, O'Brien JG, Gadd MG, Ristuccia J, Wallace DL, and Gregory M, Massachusetts Advocates for Children Trauma and Learning Policy Initiative, *Helping Traumatized Children Learn: Supportive school environments for Children traumatized by family violence*, Massachusetts Advocates for Children, Boston, MA, 2005.
34. Wolpow R, Johnson MM, Hertel R, and Kincaid SO, *The Heart of Learning and Teaching: Compassion, Resiliency, and Academic Success*, Washington State Office of Superintendent of Public Instruction (OSPI) Compassionate Schools, 2009.

10
The End

Were it possible for us to see further than our knowledge reaches, and yet a little way beyond the outworks of our own divinings, perhaps we would endure our sadnesses with greater confidence than our joys—For they are the moments when something new has entered into us, something unknown; our feelings grow mute in sly perplexity, everything in us withdraws, a stillness resumes, and the new, which no one knows, stands in the midst of it and is silent. (1)

I have heard it told that when Beethoven played his "Moonlight Sonata" at a house concert for the first time, someone came up afterward and asked, "What does this music mean?"

"I'll tell you what it means," Beethoven said. Then he sat down and played it again. (2)

Introduction

I'm finding it as impossible as Beethoven did to "tell" you what this book means, or to figure out how it should end, or even to know what it has said to you. I also can't, at the moment, "play it again"—it has lived underneath the ground of my being for so long that it is time to send it out to you. I feel inclined to approach this subject from a spiritual dimension, and from the dimension of hope.

Three Goals, Three Hopes

I hope I have accompanied some of you, at least, on a journey of sorts into the common and the unknown. What is known? People get sick, and we are tasked with prevention, cure, amelioration, and solace. What's less known and, I believe, not enough taught, is that early trauma and stress play a major role in setting off and maintaining many human ailments, "physical" and "mental." We are just discovering how the brain, and its electrical, neurochemical, hormonal, and immune relations with the body, can and does participate structurally when things go right, or wrong.

Right now, rather late in my life, I am trying to learn how to ride a horse. This, it seems, involves a complex interplay of numerous muscular commands, human psychology, horse abilities and emotion, and environmental stimuli, all interacting to produce whatever it is that just happened (often pretty awkward). "Give me three takeaways from this lesson," I plead with my riding teacher. I don't always get all three, or, if I do, I find it hard to remember them much less put them into reliable use. If I get more than three, my ability to learn is definitely shot. So, I'm going to give you three "takeaways," three end points I hope you have incorporated, and wish you a good journey in your own practice of medicine.

One. We practitioners have become accustomed to knowing we don't have enough time to spend with each patient, certainly not enough to enter into the depths described in prior chapters. I believe this is true. We do, however, have some agency and can most likely create *some* leeway with our appointed time with people. The reality is, however, that whatever interval we do have with someone, our time is always limited. Therefore, I have tried to stress the need to sharpen our listening and observational skills, so that we can quickly come to take in what is said, what is not said, and what is implied. What takes place in our body, in our patient's body, and between us—practitioner and patient? This is all information we can use. By trial and error, one must also sharpen one's intuitive skills, to sense when the time is right to speak, when to say nothing, and when to let our body respond. Following the patient's narrative, asking a curious question, raising one's eyebrows, sharing one's thoughts—none of this takes inordinate amounts of time, and it may lead the two of you into new, rewarding territory. A doctor's taking a little risk with a question will be noticed by a patient. It may inspire her to do the same.

Two. Judgment and control are two abilities we all labor for years to achieve. In working with a patient who has a trauma history, however, the work entails setting these hard-won skills aside. Barring any life-threatening behavior, we have to allow the patient maximum control over his narrative and destiny. This patient has, in essence, been held down, then beaten, raped, denigrated, ignored. Attempted control by others is experienced as a repetition of these crimes. Your patient has put himself back together as best he can, and talking about these events, even becoming aware of them, may shake his sense of trust in you, stability within himself, and the veracity of his words. What to do as the truth comes out? The patient must decide. Furthermore, judgment, in the sense of having an opinion, a reaction, a label for this patient, must be banished from the room. "Clinical judgment"—important, and so necessary—can too easily morph into pigeonholing, reacting, and blaming the patient, three things that will shut down a healing relationship faster than you can blink. Trauma clients already feel an immense weight of shame from within themselves, their abusers, and from our societies. They cannot and should not receive it from us.

Three. Some of our trauma patients will choose various types of therapies—groups, spiritual pursuits, individual therapists, books, self-healing methods—and many will not. Whether or not they do, you as a medical healer have an important role to play, both as an abiding witness and as a wise physician. For one thing, many such patients' illnesses may have a basis in trauma stressors. In addition, you are the person who, along with the patient, is chosen to receive the body's signals about this history. Finally, it's not so much what you do that makes the difference; what matters is how you are, and how you build, sustain, and understand your relationships with these patients and with all patients. The importance both of witnessing a trauma patient's struggle and your acts of simple acceptance and recognition cannot be underestimated.

One hope I have is that I have accompanied you well on this path of inquiry which may change how you choose to be with trauma patients. A second hope is that you have come to understand that once we relax a need to control our patients and their trajectory, we gain power and respect. Our power comes from our willingness to hear and partake of what has happened to them. Power comes from the sharing of the story. It comes from listening with intuition, beginning to understand, and also from not knowing and admitting it.

A third hope has to do with our many roles. I hope that those of us who lead, or who interact with our communities, will be emboldened to speak effectively for those who have been silenced. I hope that those who have responsibility for the education of our next generations of clinicians will put the issues included here on the "must be covered" list. I hope that those of us who do basic and translational research will delve more thoroughly into brain and body science. Given the prevalence of violence in our society, I hope that those who concern themselves with "outcomes" will realize the value of time invested in all of these endeavors.

We're near the end of this book now, and the words "the end" reflect my childish desire to announce it. As a doctor, I am only too aware of life's endings, often in the midst of a life and not so welcome. Death has the ability to march up and take over our human intentions. There is not always a next visit. Then too, many of our relationships with patients end before their life is over. People move, need someone different, need to run away, or just change insurances. We work toward understanding what we are to do, but the opportunity to do it may slip away from us. Finally, in dealing with past violence, I don't think we ever do reach an end. We can hope for some more wholeness for our patients, some reintegration with life, some ability to care for self and future generations. We can aspire to play a part in that process. But we can never undo what has been done. Like so much in the pursuit of health, prevention is the best medicine.

Sheila and Amber will illustrate.

Sheila

I saw Sheila for over 20 years, late in her life. She was referred by her second husband, already my patient for many years. She had been married in her teens and had three daughters, one of whom became a lawyer. Eventually, when the children were grown, her first husband died. Sheila smoked heavily for many years, enough to have now caused COPD.

Sheila had remarried by the time I met her, a man (my patient) on whom she became financially and then physically dependent, due to the onset of severe hearing loss and progression of breathing difficulties. Patient, husband, and doctor weathered the advancing deafness, severe chronic lung disease, development of breast cancer and its treatment, and a life-threatening pulmonary embolus, all of which Sheila survived. She spent most days sitting at home, alone.

Early in the second marriage, it became clear to Sheila that her new husband was a pedophile and was having affairs with men as well. Had I already known all of this? Somehow, my memory fails me. I think I had heard some of it, but it's all murky—dissociated. In any case, Sheila did not feel she could leave her husband, but she became increasingly "disgusted" with his presence. As she got to know me, dissatisfaction, despair with the marriage, and dependence were themes of every visit.

I treated her husband for over 30 years for chronic lung disease, severe complications of cardiovascular disease, secondary syphilis, and other intermittent ailments. By the time I was caring for Sheila, I knew about his predilections for secretive, furtive exploits with men and boys. I never asked about his childhood or how he became driven in this way. Of course, I strongly suspect now that he must also have been a victim of childhood abuse.

Sheila revealed her own past trauma to me, triggered one day by her becoming aware that her husband was having a new affair with a male neighbor in a downstairs apartment. As we talked about this, she was reminded of her father, who had been murderously violent with her mother and had gone to jail because of this for some years, but returned home to rape Sheila repeatedly in her early adolescence. As usual, she recounted her narrative of past and present in a cynical, distant tone of voice. She "didn't care." Yet, Sheila kept bringing things up. I felt like she was a million miles away, and breathing down my neck, at the same time.

Terribly ashamed of her husband and, I suspected, of herself, she made things even more confusing by periodically noting his attention to her, his occasionally thoughtful acts, and his general caring for her in her increasing infirmity. In fact, in separate visits, her husband would approach me with a smile on his face, "hat in hand," solicitous about Sheila, her depression, her shortness of breath, her unhappiness.

Sheila complained frequently, bitterly, and in a sarcastic monotone about her husband's infidelity, his preoccupation with boys and men; about her fears of catching something from him (she had withdrawn from sexual activity with him before I met her, shortly after the marriage); about her embarrassment. Visits would then end as she recounted the fact that she had saved some money that she intended to leave to her grandchildren as a surprise, which she believed they would use to make themselves a better life than she had had.

As their doctor, I felt helpless to affect this cycle. Any and all suggestions to Sheila were dismissed as impossible, and truly I felt no way out of Sheila's dilemma. After many years of treatment, she abruptly fired me and went off to one, then another, then a third female physician in the next three years. Her last months were spent in an assisted living facility.

Her husband, having refused a defibrillator for his advanced cardiac disease, died of "natural causes" some months after Sheila left the practice. He actually hoped to die suddenly and painlessly, and he did. Sheila found him dead in bed. He was always grateful for my "good care."

I used to dread Sheila's visits. I knew what to do about her COPD, her cancer, her clot prevention, but I felt under-powered to deal with both her present and her past. Sometimes, I felt angry at her for complaining and never changing. Other times, I wondered to myself why *anyone* would marry a pedophile. I wondered if bitterness kept her going, and what that was like. I only briefly questioned how I had provided the "last straw" that caused her to leave the practice. Although I knew whom she went to see, I never inquired about her well-being. I let myself lose track of her.

In short, I felt Sheila was in charge and that I was her victim during our visits. Her illnesses, disability, and her previous experiences had locked us both in the present situation. I could not think of what to do, so I just endured her visits and took care of her bodily issues. Judgment on my part covered over my helplessness. I didn't know why she came to see me. I could not think of how to be helpful. At one point, both husband and wife were in the hospital at the same time, and she threatened not to go home with him. I felt vaguely hopeful for her, and frightened for her, too. But as always, she relented and returned to her lonely living room.

The End with Sheila

Sheila seemed to have learned the lessons of childhood trauma very well. Her father's voice: "You are helpless in front of me, no one can 'hear' you, you do not deserve better, you will feel this shame forever." Nicotine addiction, its short-term boosts and long-term consequences, and her "choices" of spouses led to further traumas, disability, confinement, and progressively fewer options for living her life in freedom.

During the years I cared for Sheila, I didn't know anything about the "trauma quadrangle" (see Chapter 5), much less about how to get out of one, about how not to be a rescuer, for instance. I was the prisoner of my own reactions to her situation. I worry now that her departure had to do with her perceptions of my unspoken judgment of her ("why would anyone marry a pedophile?") or my unexplained irritation. It could also have related to the dilemma for her, and me, that my caring for both her and her husband posed. Or maybe she got sick of powerlessness and fired me because it was something she *could do*.

As I review Sheila's situation, I also now understand that she was coping by dissociating, and that it had enveloped me as well. One key to understanding this comes in recalling her sarcastic, monotonous recounting of terrible events, both past and present. The "real" Sheila, who had dealt with the unspeakable, sent the sarcastic, contemptuous "Greek chorus" to recite to me and my ilk—whoever was "in the audience."

Philip Bromberg writes for therapists of the dilemma this poses by "quoting" a hypothetical dissociating patient:

> I'm here because I'm in trouble, but the trouble I'm in is not something I need rescuing from, even though it may look that way. However, I fully expect you to try to "cure" me and, I'm prepared to defeat you. I don't have an illness, I *am* my illness, and I won't let you cure me of being who I am. (3)

A further conceptualization. Sheila, her husband, and I were enveloped in the experiences of each of our "good me, bad me, and not-me"—personae by which Harry Stack Sullivan first elaborated his theory of dissociation as a way of living with early, horrendous, incomprehensible experience. The "good me and bad me" are conscious, according to Sullivan. "Not-me" is not conscious. "The not-me is literally the organization of experience with significant people that has been subjected to such intense anxiety . . . that it was impossible for the then relatively rudimentary person to make any sense of that experience.

The experiences stored in 'not-me' are connected with sickening, sudden, paralyzing anxiety and by 'uncanny emotions.' "

My medical doctoring, Sheila's saving for grandchildren, and the husband's seeking care for his wife were all "good me" personas. My relief at her departure, the husband's sexual adventures, and Sheila's sarcastic dismissal of her husband were the "bad me" elements. The "not-me" (dissociated set of feelings and memory) is, according to Sullivan, hinted at by the "uncanny emotions" of awe (husband at the power of doctoring), dread (me of Sheila's visits), loathing (Sheila's "disgusted"), and horror (the stories, which we all mostly ignored) (4). The appearance of any of these, in a clinical dyad or a family system, can be a clue to the alert practitioner that a past serious transgression against one's patient—some sort of evil, to someone anyway—may be lurking underneath the story as told.

A consultation about how I felt about Sheila might have helped us both. For instance, over the years I've participated in various groups blending internal medicine and a psychiatric provider—some self-styled as "Balint" groups (5). In them, we have presented "problem patients"—mostly, patients whose words and actions provoke problematic emotions and responses in us, or people whose behavior we do not understand or like very much. Such groups talk about hating patients and being bamboozled by them. The groups explore themselves. They strategize about next steps. They employ mutual positive regard. Such groups can cheer us on, nurture courage, and provide options and self-understanding. The help of interested, educated others can sometimes uncover that which escapes us.

"We all hover at different distances between knowing and not knowing about trauma, caught between the compulsion to complete the process of knowing and the inability or fear of doing so. It is the nature of trauma to elude our knowledge because of both defense and deficit . . . trauma overwhelms and defeats our capacity to organize it" (6).

I was glad to learn that Sheila spent the end of her days in an assisted living facility, not reliant on a spouse who shamed and frightened her (as well as cared for her). By the time I met her, in her older age, could we have done anything more useful together? I don't know. I do regret that, as a relative youngster in medicine back then, I knew so little about parts of the self and could not recognize that Sheila's "bad me" challenged my "not-me." There are far too many Sheilas in the world, their lives severely impaired by the physical and mental sequelae of childhood sexual abuse and other trauma.

Amber

Amber, in her 40s, first consulted me after entering her menopause surgically. From the first, she displayed an open and frank, healthy-feeling style. She'd grown up in another part of the country but after college there, had traveled internationally seeking service and adventure. After her return, she attended graduate school, then moved to our area. Did she miss her home? Not a bit—"too racist" for her. On my practice's then standard, obtuse form asking about marriage, she wrote boldly, "I'm gay and not living with anyone now." Amber seemed comfortable with herself, open to a new person as a medical provider, and capable of some risk. This was the sort of person I looked forward to seeing.

Amber told me she was seeing a therapist who specialized in grown children with alcoholic parents. Her father had been, and several sibs were, afflicted with the disease of alcoholism. She wanted to get on a more regular mammogram program. All of this seemed like healthy housekeeping in young middle age. She did complain of chronic vaginal itching, which she thought was related to a yeast infection. Her general and pelvic exams were completely normal, and I wondered if this symptom signaled another problem "itching" to be revealed. However, vaginal culture did show a few yeast, and I advised treatment and regular prophylaxis. I had the feeling that some as-yet cloudy "thing" had been a call for her to pay more attention to herself, or perhaps attention of a different kind. In addition, we note now that after taking care of health maintenance issues, her vagina spoke up.

Over the next two to three years, her mother and a sister died, menopausal symptoms emerged, and she felt conflicted about estrogen but seemed to need it. She changed careers to a "more peaceful" occupation and then told me that she was "actively healing" from her father's alcoholism as well as from sexual abuse by father and uncle. She had only recently discovered the abuse while doing hypnotherapy with a local psychologist. Amber's "activity" in healing connotes her cooperation, invitation, or command of the process. Not a victim of her past, she sees herself as moving the healing along. She's not asking for or needing my help; she is keeping the sources of her help to herself. She's the captain of her own ship. Amber doesn't tell me about the abuse until she tells me about her healing. We understand a different reason why she might want to be far from home. Also, another facet of herself is "out." Neither of us seemed inclined to go into details. Was this an error? Was I reading her signals correctly? Was I too stunned by this ugliness in Amber's past to take in what she had just said? Does this "stunning" process mirror her original experiences of trauma?

Amber went on to have a breast lumpiness evaluation (negative), and concerns over a vaginal bump (was estrogen the culprit?) (no pathology). There was an interlude with a trusted partner covering my patients while I was out of the country, where she again displayed her open style and her ability to "engage" warmly with new professionals. She had an uneventful laparoscopic cholecystectomy. This all occurred over a period of several years.

Nine years into our relationship, she came for a general exam. In her chart, I wrote "She continues in therapy with Dr. (X) with whom she has been working on her tendency to chose as partners people who are abusive. In the last relationship, which ended five years ago, she thought *she* was becoming abusive. She is concluding that she best not be in a relationship, although this is a painful loss for her." A colonoscopy had shown adenomatous polyps, and she would need regular surveillance. This body intrusion had not troubled her unduly. There was another discussion about risks/benefits of hormones. Amber continued to share openly her successes and shortcomings as a mature human being. I, meanwhile, wondered again if I should, or should have, asked her for more details about the traumatic events that had happened to her in her family. Was this a shortcoming in our relationship? I let the question slide.

Years passed. Amber began to tire of her occupation. She gave up estrogen, after many years of use, without a problem. She gave up her administrative duties. Again, in her chart: "She has had a variety of failed relationships. She has decided that she's better off alone. She keeps making 'bad choices,' people that she takes care of, and then leave her. She thinks she can't get over it, even after years of therapy." She looked and felt very well and had a completely normal exam.

The following year she had resigned her position, though remaining active in a few aspects of her work. She was enjoying the "soul rest" of retirement. For the first time in years, however, she once more complained of some vaginal itching and, this time, a change in the appearance of her labia minora. She appeared to have some sort of labial dystrophy—not an infection. She was referred for a biopsy, which revealed lichen sclerosis et atrophicus—a soft tissue/skin disease of the genital area which can occur in both men and women, which causes atrophy of the genital area and itching. The cause is "unknown," and the disease is chronic.

It seems that the "first word" will also be the "last word." Amber's vagina will never stop speaking. Scaer's (7) work on the psychophysiology of trauma postulates that the experience(s) result in encapsulated or embedded autonomic arousal. One's autonomic nervous system, conditioned to respond to threat by flight, fight, or freeze, is vulnerable to never working correctly after episodes of deadly threat. Circulatory changes appropriate for the threatening situation thereafter respond inappropriately, chronically, and autonomously to minor stimuli, creating via the circulation excessive or insufficient supply of nutrients and removal of waste metabolites, causing organ damage. Could this mechanism underlie the atrophy and nerve stimulation of lichen sclerosis? (What role did stopping estrogen have, as well?)

Summing up the situation, I gathered my courage and asked Amber directly about what specifically had happened in her past. She looked shocked, and then, with her usual forthrightness, she began. When she was seven or eight, her father's brother had returned from wartime military service and found himself homeless, so lived with them for some time. She now felt he had had PTSD. He repeatedly enticed and threatened her, and perhaps at least one of her sisters, into experiences involving oral and genital penetration. Her parents never knew. (She did not mention anything on this day about her father, even though she had implicated him previously). Later, as a young adult, one night during an outdoor education experience she was violently raped by the sole male instructor while alone in her tent, perched next to a mountainous cliff. He molested her viciously while expressing his hatred of all women. She was convinced that he meant to kill her by throwing her off the cliff when he was done. She expressed absolutely nothing, but lay still, instinctively "feeling" this was the safest thing for her to do (the "freeze"). Eventually, he left the tent. The next morning they got up, ate together, and she relied on his expertise, which he freely gave, to get down off the mountain. As with her uncle and her parents, no words were spoken about what had happened. Amber had never related these experiences to any medical provider.

We continued for several years more with pretty routine care. At some point we discussed this book project, about which she was quite positive, including the possibility that her story might be included. Amber eventually decided to move closer to younger family out of state, thinking of care she might need as she aged. As a parting gift she brought me a piece of her work which she thought might help me in writing this book.

The End with Amber

As with many patients in mobile America, my long relationship with Amber came to an end when she needed to move. Her life will have other chapters, but she and I are done. She had the luck and privilege to be able to engage in helpful, long-term therapy, and to benefit from it. It took her time, energy, and likely a good chunk of her disposable income. Many people do not have those options.

Despite Amber's access to treatment, her traumas left her with an inability to negotiate a safe love relationship for herself. As well, she has developed a medically unexplained (though fairly common) syndrome, which as of now is incurable. The lichen sclerosis may or may not have anything to do with what happened to her, though it is hard to write it off as unrelated. She has had to mourn her aloneness (while still preserving a bit of hope) and to live with a vagina that will never be quiet. She will always need to listen to and take care of it.

Amber was never moved to "disclose" to me. I wouldn't call her statements about therapy "hints." They felt to me like "way closing" not "way opening," like background scenery to our time together. I had to ask her, and she was clearly shaken, though emotionally prepared to talk. Had I not seemed trustworthy enough? Had she and I unwittingly subscribed to the developed world's mind–body split in medicine? Was she protecting me, or herself, from the feelings associated with memory? Would an earlier disclosure and then work have changed her outcome? Amber and I experienced many moments of great satisfaction in our relationship with each other, and her health was generally very good. But I am left with such questions.

"Good Clinicians Are Strange Instruments"

I don't think I can do any better at the end than repeating the thoughts of internist Dr. Eric Cassell:

> It cannot be said too often that in learning to communicate effectively . . . listening, really listening, is as important as talking. Part of listening is learning to be completely open in the presence of the patient . . . (as if) there were a door to the inside of you . . . and you consciously opened it so the patient would flow into you. . . . This stance is not something you do as much as something you are. Properly done, no one but you will know exactly what is happening, not even the patients. (8)

Dr. Cassell was talking about helping patients suffering from illness and approaching death. His words, however, apply to the suffering caused by childhood abuse and neglect, which engenders its own illnesses, as we have seen, and both psychic and physical death. I will repeat that ongoing awareness of trauma and its prevalence must precede this openness. As well, clinicians must prepare, and be properly prepared, for the effects of openness to patients' feelings, stories, and behaviors, on themselves. Knowledge and emotional education are both important.

We are left with what we do and do not, and can and cannot do. We cannot "cure" a person of a traumatic past as if it were a strep throat or breast cancer. Nor can we be perfect communicators on all occasions. We can, however, aspire to be present to patients, acknowledging their truths and realities, and taking in their adaptations and aspirations. We can keep in mind their stories, and their wounds, as we tend and try to mend their bodies. We can hold all of these realities together for people even if, for them, they embody separate states of being. We can do this even if we do not understand them ourselves, which we must humbly admit must often be the case.

I would emphasize to all healers the critical importance of their witness function. Practicing medicine properly allows for a privileged, intimate relationship. In it, patients can share their entire stories, and selves, and clinicians grow in skill, knowledge, awareness, and empathy. Being a witness allows patients to trade the safety of aloneness and an incomplete self for relatedness, and for taking the risks which accompany growth. Witnessing skills are something that can be taught and learned by present and future practitioners, if we put our hearts and minds to it.

References

1. From *Letters to a Young Poet* by Rainer Maria Rilke, translated by M.D. Herter Norton. Copyright 1934, 1954 by W.W. Norton & Company, renewed © 1962, 1982 by M.D. Herter Norton. Used by permission of W.W. Norton and Company, Inc., 1993.
2. Kidd SM, *First Light, Early Inspirational Writings*, Penguin Books, 2007. Copyright © 2007 by Sue Monk Kidd, LLC.
3. Bromberg P, *Standing in the Spaces, Essays on Clinical Process, Trauma and Dissociation*, 207–208, The Analytic Press, 1998.
4. Sullivan HS, *The Interpersonal Theory of Psychiatry*, pp. 314–317, WW Norton, 1953.
5. Crossman S, "Investing in each other: Balint groups and the patient-doctor relationship," *Virtual Mentor* 14(7): 551–554, 2012.
6. Laub D and Auerhohn NC, "Knowing and not knowing, massive psychic trauma: Forms of traumatic memory," *International Journal of Psychoanalysis* 74:287–302, 1993.
7. Scaer R, *The Trauma Spectrum, Hidden Wounds and Human Resiliency*, WW Norton, 2005.
8. Cassell EJ, *The Nature of Suffering and the Goals of Medicine*, 2nd edition, Oxford University Press, 2004.

Index

For the benefit of digital users, indexed terms that span two pages (e.g., 52–53) may, on occasion, appear on only one of those pages.

A
abdominal pain
Marta (case study), 76–82
Peg (case study), 154–56
abusive power, 86–89
ACEs (adverse childhood experiences), 108–9
ACE score, 108–9
ACOG (American College of Obstetrics and Gynecology), 3–4, 18–19
ACTH, 38–39
addiction
Darlene (case study), 122–26
denial of, 64
and PTSD, 48, 49
stigma in medical care, 106–7
Adler, H. M., 166–67
adverse childhood experiences (ACEs), 108–9, 146
affective impulses, alterations in regulation of, 35
Alaggia, R., 17–18, 162–63
alcoholism
and ACEs, 108–9
Amber (case study), 205–8
medical understanding of, 106
Rosita (case study), 119–22
as self-injury, 108
alexithymia, 143
Alpert, E. J., 162
altered perceptions
Marta (case study), 76–82
overview, 65
Amber (case study), 205–8
ambivalent alliance, 140–41
American College of Obstetrics and Gynecology (ACOG), 3–4, 18–19
amnesia
in complex PTSD, 35
dissociative, 33, 35
traumatic, 65, 82–83
amygdalae, 40
Anda, R., 146–47
Angela (case study), 167–73
anger
and abusive power, 88
in complex PTSD, 35
and doctor-patient relationships, 165
and self-harm, 114, 118
anorexia, 111–16, 118–19
anterior cingulate gyrus, 40, 128–29, 151–52
arm pain, 51–59
Armsworth, M. W., 192
arousal symptoms, 33, 45–47
arterial insufficiency, 51–59
atrocity, 88–89
attachment
and orbitofrontal cortex, 41
and PTSD risk, 42, 44–45
and self-harm, 116–17
attention, alterations in, 35
attuned listening, 15, 34
autonomic arousal, embedded, 206
avoidant symptoms, 32, 45–47, 51

B
Baddeley, J. L., 20
Bala, M., 163–64
Balint groups, 204
Battaglia, T., 184
Best, D., 129–30
bias, physician, 163, 164
biological substrates of PTSD, 38–41
biopsychosocial model, 153–54, 158
blame, release from, 25, 26
body, impact of trauma on
Bonnie (case study), 145–46
chaos, 144–46
disclosure through body, 22–23
Gabe (case study), 26–28

body, impact of trauma on (*cont.*)
integrating knowledge of abuse into care, 152–56
models for understanding, 141–44
Nina (case study), 23–26
obesity as somatization disorder, 146–48
overview, 135–37
Peg (case study), 154–56
Sharon (case study), 150–52
speech of the body, 137–41
treatment approaches, 148–52, 157–59
body language of providers, 15
body memory, 22–23
Bolen, R. M., 9–10, 12
Bonds, D. E., 181
Bonhomme, J., 127
Bonnie (case study), 145–46
boundaries, problems with, 50
Bowlby, J., 42
brachial aneurysm, 51–59
brain
and ACEs, 146–47
and dissociation, 73–82
and MUS, 143–44
stress response in, 38–41
and substance abuse, 128–29
breast cancer and reconstruction, 167–73
Breslau short screening scale for PTSD, 46
Briere, J., 36
Broadbent, E., 143
Bromberg, P., 203
Brown, R. J., 142
bulimia, 108
burnout, 185–86

C
cancellations of appointments, 98–102
Cassell, E. J., 138–39, 208
catastrophizing symptoms, 143
CBT (cognitive behavioral therapy), 25, 26
cerebral cortex, 38–41
cervical ribs, 51–59
chaos, 144–46
Chen, W., 193
chest pain
Elora (case study), 51–59
Sharon (case study), 150–52
Chico, L. S., 96–97
chief complaints, paying attention to, 117
child abuse specialists, 178
childhood maltreatment, 128–29
childhood sexual abuse. *See also* disclosure of abuse
abusive power, 86–89
Amber (case study), 205–8
Angela (case study), 167–73
Bonnie (case study), 145–46
common symptoms in adult survivors of, 3–6
definitions and awareness of, 10–12
Gabe (case study), 67–71
and health care, 50
and MUS, 152–56
Oliver (case study), 4–8
Peg (case study), 154–56
professional response to, 8–10
and PTSD risk, 42, 43, 44
reasons for not seeking help after, 162–63
under-reporting of, 177–78
Rosita (case study), 119–22
Sheila (case study), 201–4
and substance abuse, 48
trust, building, 91–93
child protection team (CPT), 193
child sexual abuse accommodation syndrome, 163–64
chronic pain, 122–26
Chung, S., 191
Clarke, D. M., 138
clinical judgment, 162, 199–200
clinical leadership, 94–95
coaches, sexual assault by, 43
coercion, 16, 87, 180–81
cognitive behavioral therapy (CBT), 25, 26
coherent narrative, developing, 149–50
colonoscopy, 6, 7
combat veterans. *See* military trauma
communication. *See also* disclosure of abuse
through cutting, 114–15
written, 78
complexity theory, 166–67
complex PTSD
Clyde (case study), 36–37
Elora (case study), 51–59
general discussion, 34–36
concentration camp experiences, 185
Confronting Chronic Neglect (Institute of Medicine report), 8, 99
consciousness, alterations in, 35
control, 199–200
controlled identification, 185
co-opting of providers, 188–89

coronary disease, 110–11, 150–52
corpus callosum, 39, 75–76
corticotropin release factor (CRF), 38–39
cortisol responses, 38–39, 143–44
CPT (child protection team), 193
cutting
  communication function of, 114–15
  feelings behind, 111–14
  Linnea (case study), 111–13, 115–16
  professional response to, 117–19
  and secure attachment, 116–17
  stigma, 109–11
cystoscopy, 69–71, 73, 78

D
Darlene (case study), 122–26, 127–28
declarative memory, 74
defense mechanism, dissociation as, 64–71
defensive styles, 185
denial, 8–10, 64, 185
dental extractions, 76–77, 82
depression
  and childhood maltreatment, 128
  Nina (case study), 23–26
  Olivia (case study), 187–88
  and PTSD, 48
  Rosita (case study), 119–22
  Susan (case study), 33–34
  Val (case study), 98–102
detachment, 33, 45–47
diabetes mellitus, 154–56
disclosure of abuse
  among professionals, 187–88
  beneficial, 182–83
  communication strategies for, 181–82
  desired practices, 21–25
  enabling, 20–25
  Gabe (case study), 26–28
  importance of, 28
  limitations of language, 50
  Nina (case study), 23–26
  overview, 14–15
  and PTSD risk, 44–45
  reasons preventing victims from, 162–63
  research on, 17–20
  of sexual trauma, 50
  special considerations, 15–16
Disorders of Extreme Stress, not otherwise specified (DESNOS), 34–37
dissociation
  brain and, 73–82
  as defense mechanism, 64–71
  Gabe (case study), 67–71
  Marta (case study), 76–82
  and medical practice, 66–71
  overview, 63
  during physical exams, 100–1
  recognition of, 71–73, 82–83
  Sharon (case study), 150–52
  Sheila (case study), 201–4
dissociative amnesia, 33, 35
DMSO infusions, 78–79
doctor-patient relationship
  Angela (case study), 167–73
  in complex PTSD, 35
  impact of disclosure on, 28
  overview, 161
  with trauma survivor, 162–73
domestic violence
  and clinical judgment, 162
  integrated practice, 182–84
  medical training in, 177–79
  Olivia (case study), 187–88
  personal issues for health care providers, 184–88
  practice regarding, 179–82
  and provider gender, 186–87
  recognizing and reporting of abuse, 188–90
  trauma-informed systems of care, 190–95
dorsal vagal complex, 75
duplicity, 88–89, 91

E
eating disorders
  and ACEs, 108–9
  Linnea (case study), 111–13, 115–16
  as self-injury, 108
  stigma in medical care, 107
Ebell, M., 46–47
education about violence, 8–10
Egnew, T. R., 167
elder abuse education, 178–79
Elora (case study), 51–59, 66–67, 103
empathy, 157, 166–67, 179, 192
empowerment, 90, 94–95
enactments
  Angela (case study), 167–73
  overview, 165–66
Engel, G., 153–54
Epstein, R., 140
explicit memory, 74, 142–43

extrafamilial abuse, 12, 18

F
"false memory" syndrome, 45
fear of rejection, 17, 20–21
Felitti, V. J., 108–9, 147–48
fight response, 74–75
Filipas, H., 44
Finkelhor, D., 12
flashbacks, 32, 40, 65, 82–83, 120–21
flight response, 74–75
Forgash, C., 184
freeze discharge, 75
freeze response, 74–75
Friedman, L. S., 19
functional illness, 49–50

G
Gabe (case study), 26–28, 67–71, 72–73
Gabriel, G. M., 193
gang rape, 88–89
gender
 building trust, 91
 prevalence of abuse by, 12
 provider response to domestic abuse, 186–88
 trauma-informed system, 192–93
genital concerns
 Amber (case study), 205–8
 Gabe (case study), 26–28, 67–71
 Marta (case study), 76–82
 repeated focus on, 27
Gerber, M. R., 183
Gibbons, J., 192
Gilligan, J., 1–2
GI symptoms
 Elora (case study), 56–57
 Marta (case study), 77
 and MUS, 153–54
 Oliver (case study), 4–8
 Peg (case study), 154–56
"good me, bad me, and not-me" personae, 203–4
Gordon, A., 129
Greenleaf, R. K., 95
guilt, 20–21, 33, 35, 185
Gutmanis, I., 179–80

H
headaches
 Darlene (case study), 122–26
 and terrible narratives, 149
health care. *See* medical care
hemispheric activity in PTSD, 40
Herman, J., 94, 130–31, 164–65
hippocampus, 40–41, 74, 146–47
Hoppe, K. D., 185
hospitalizations, 48–50
humility, 104
hypermnesia, 65, 82–83
hypervigilance, 33, 45–47
hypothalamic pituitary (HPA) axis, 143–44, 146–47

I
implicit memory, 22–23, 74, 142–43, 151–52
incoherent narrative, 149–50
injury to self, 107–9
insomnia
 Gabe (case study), 68
 Rosita (case study), 119–22
Institute of Medicine, 8, 99
insula, 41
interpersonal relations following trauma, 44
interstitial cystitis, 78–81
intimate partner violence (IPV), 177, 180–81, 186–87
intimidation of providers, 189
intrusive symptoms, 32, 36, 45–47, 50
intuitive skills, 199
irritable bowel syndrome, 154–56

J
Jenny, C., 189
Jones, J., 36
judgment, 162, 199–200

K
Kartha, A., 48
Kimerling, R., 45–46

L
Lang, A., 47
language disturbance, 114–15
language in disclosure, limitations of, 50
Lanius, R., 39–41
lateralization of brain function, 40
leadership, clinical, 94–95
Leahy, T., 43
learned helplessness, 36
Leserman, J., 153
lichen sclerosis, 206, 207

Liebschutz, J., 182–83
limbic system, 39
Linnea (case study), 111–16
listening skills
  attuned, 15
  in integrated practice, 184
  and medical power, 90, 104
  need to sharpen, 199
  physician openness, 208
  treating MUS, 148–50
low social recognition, 186
Lubman, D., 129–30

M

Magana, H., 149–50
Mammen, G., 191–92
Marta (case study), 76–82
Massachusetts trauma-informed school manual, 194–95
maternal deprivation, 39
McNally, R., 44
medial prefrontal cortex, 40
medical care
  childhood sexual abuse awareness, 10–12
  and dissociation, 66–71
  Oliver (case study), 4–8
  professional response to childhood trauma, 8–10
  and PTSD, 48–50, 59–61
  symptoms of trauma, 3–8
medically unexplained symptoms (MUS)
  Angela (case study), 167–73
  Bonnie (case study), 145–46
  and chaos, 144–46
  integrating knowledge of abuse into care, 152–56
  models for, 141–44
  obesity as somatization disorder, 146–48
  overview, 135–37
  Peg (case study), 154–56
  Sharon (case study), 150–52
  speech of the body, 137–41
  treatment models, 148–52, 157–59
medical power, 89–93
medical training in trauma, 177–79
memory alteration, 65, 82–83
mental health professional, abuse by, 187–88
military trauma
  and abusive power, 86–87, 88–89
  PC-PTSD screening device for, 46–47
  PTSD in, 40–41, 44, 48
mind, 74–75
Mollica, R. F., 184
Monahan, K., 184
moral complexity of trauma, 44
Morrissey, J. P., 191
Murphy, S. B., 20
MUS. *See* medically unexplained symptoms
mutual alliance, 140–41

N

naming illness, 158
narcotic abuse, 122–26
narratives, 149–50
negative cognitions, 32–33, 45–47
negative social reactions, 44
negotiation
  Elora (case study), 102–4
  Val (case study), 98–102
Nemeroff, C., 39
neocortex, 39
neuroanatomy
  and ACEs, 146–47
  of dissociation, 73–82
  and MUS, 143–44
  of stress response, 38–41
  and substance abuse, 128–29
Nicolaidis, C., 179
Nina (case study), 23–26
Noether, C. D., 191
non-alliance, 140–41
nonverbal pattern, 41
Norman, D. A., 143
not-me persona, 203–4
numbing, 65–66

O

obesity
  Bonnie (case study), 145–46
  Nina (case study), 23–26
  Peg (case study), 154–56
  as somatization disorder, 146–48
  Val (case study), 98–102
observational skills, 199
obstetric practice, 18–19, 21–25
Olde Hartman, T. C., 140–41
Olivia (case study), 187–88
opioid prescriptions, 122–27
orbitofrontal cortex, 41
overdose deaths, 126–27
over-identification, 185
over-referral, avoiding, 158

oxycodone, 122–27

P

pain
  Darlene (case study), 122–26
  Elora (case study), 51–59
  Marta (case study), 76–82
  overview, 82–83
  Peg (case study), 154–56
  Sharon (case study), 150–52
panic, 65
panic attacks, 23–26, 68
PC-PTSD screening instrument, 47
Peg (case study), 154–56
penile hemorrhage, 69–70
Percocet addiction, 122–26
perpetrators
  abusive power, 16, 86–89
  alterations in perception of, 35
  and PTSD risk, 43
  victim triangle, 96–97
Peters, S., 141, 148–49
physical abuse
  Marta (case study), 76–82
  under-reporting of, 177–78
physical exams, avoidance of, 98–102
physician response
  to dissociation, 71–73, 82–83
  to MUS, 140–41, 144
  to trauma survivor, 162–73
  trust, building, 91–93
Plakun, E. M., 165–66
PMPS (Preventive Medical Psychiatry Service), 193
Point of Care (PC) guideline for PTSD screening, 46–47
post-traumatic stress disorder (PTSD)
  biological substrates of, 38–41
  caring for persons with, 59–61
  characteristic behaviors in, 50–58
  Clyde (case study), 36–37
  complex PTSD, 34–37
  defined, 31–33
  Elora (case study), 51–59
  and health care, 48–50
  overview, 30–31
  risk factors for, 42–45
  screening for, 45–47
  Susan (case study), 33–34
power and control
  abusive power, 86–89
  empowerment, 94–95
  medical power, 89–93, 200
  other negotiations, 102–4
  overview, 85–86
  survivor response to powerlessness, 97–98
  trust, 91–93
  Val (case study), 98–102
  victim triangle, 96–97
powerlessness, 86–89, 90, 97–98
precipitating events, 142–43
pregnancy, 18–19, 21–25
Pretty, G., 43
prevalence of child sexual abuse, 11–12
Preventive Medical Psychiatry Service (PMPS), 193
procedural memory, 74
professional cynicism, 185
Pross, C., 185–86
psychiatrist, abuse by, 187–88
psychoeducation, 61
psychophysiology of trauma, 206
psychosocial concerns, 141, 154
PTSD. *See* post-traumatic stress disorder
pyelonephritis, 77, 82–83

R

rationalization, 185
re-attribution model, 148–49
recovery, 129–33
Reece, J., 106–7
regulation of affect, 116–17
rejection, fear of, 17, 20–21
relationship to others, alterations in, 35
reporting of abuse, 189–90
repression of memories, 18
reptilian brain, 39, 74
rescuers, in victim triangle, 96–97
respect for victims, importance of, 92–93
re-traumatization, 50, 91–92, 132
Rhodes, K. V., 181–82
rib pain, 77
Rief, W., 143
risk factors for PTSD, 42–45
Roelens, I., 180–81
Roelofs, K., 143
Rosita (case study), 119–22
Russell, D. E. H., 12
Rwanda, 96–97
Ryan, R., 188–89

S

safe place, building, 90, 117–18, 130–31
safety, 130–31
Safra Children's Hospital, in Israel, 193
Salmon, H., 141
Salmon, M. E., 71
Salmon, P., 141, 148–49
Samson, J., 128–29
SAS (supervisory attentional system), 142–43
Scaer, R., 65, 74–75, 206
Scannapieco, M., 12
Schei, E., 94–95
school manuals on trauma-informed care, 194–95
Schore, A., 40
Scott, C., 36
screaming, 66–67
screening
  for abuse, 18–19, 177–79, 180–82
  for PTSD, 45–47
secure attachment, 42, 44–45, 116–17
self-concept, 26–27
self-harm
  cutting, 109–19
  Darlene (case study), 122–26
  injury and injury to self, 107–9
  Linnea (case study), 111–13
  overview, 106–7
  reflections on recovery, 130–33
  Rosita (case study), 119–22
  substance misuse and abuse, 126–30
  understanding stigma, 107
self-perception, alterations in, 35
Seng, J. S., 21–25
servant-leadership, 95
sexual abuse. *See also* disclosure of abuse
  abusive power, 86–89
  Amber (case study), 205–8
  Angela (case study), 167–73
  Bonnie (case study), 145–46
  common symptoms in adult survivors of, 3–6
  definitions and awareness of, 10–12
  Gabe (case study), 67–71
  and health care, 50
  and male socialization, 192
  and MUS, 152–56
  Oliver (case study), 4–8
  Peg (case study), 154–56
  professional response to, 8–10
  and PTSD risk, 42, 43, 44
  reasons for not seeking help after, 162–63
  under-reporting of, 177–78
  Rosita (case study), 119–22
  Sheila (case study), 201–4
  and substance abuse, 48
  trust, building, 91–93
sexual abuse resource group, 191–92
sexuality
  Gabe (case study), 26–28, 68–71
  repeated focus on, 27–28
shadow presence, 16
Shallice, T., 143
shame
  and abusive power, 87–88
  in complex PTSD, 35
  and PTSD risk, 44
  as root of violence, 1–2
Shapiro, B., 127
Sharon (case study), 150–52
Sheila (case study), 201–4
silencing by perpetrators, 87
Singer, J. A., 20
Singh, B. S., 138
smoking
  and ACEs, 108
  Angela (case study), 167–73
  Darlene (case study), 122–26
socialization, male, 192
somatization
  Bonnie (case study), 145–46
  chaos, 144–46
  in complex PTSD, 35
  general discussion, 138–41
  humility, need for, 104
  integrating knowledge of abuse into care, 152–56
  models for, 141–44
  obesity as disorder of, 146–48
  Peg (case study), 154–56
  and PTSD, 49
  Sharon (case study), 150–52
  treatment approaches, 148–52, 157–59
Somer, E., 17
speech of the body, 137–41
Spinhoven, P., 143
stages of revelation, 20
Starling, S., 177–78
Stein, M., 47, 48
stigma
  and disclosure, 17–18, 20–21, 28
  and self-harm, 107

Stobo, J, D., 71
Stone, L., 138, 144, 157–58
Straker, G., 109–10, 114–15, 116–17
stress response
in brain, 38–41
Susan (case study), 33–34
substance abuse
and ACEs, 108–9
Darlene (case study), 122–26
denial of, 64
general discussion, 126–30
and PTSD, 48, 49
Rosita (case study), 119–22
stigma in medical care, 106–7
substance dependence, 127
Suchman, A. L., 166–67
suicide, 108–9, 114–15, 126
Sullivan, H. S., 203–4
"Summary of participant messages to providers" (Seng et al.), 21–25
supervisory attentional system (SAS), 142–43
survivors
empowerment of, 94–95
trust, building, 91–93
victim triangle, 96–97
world inhabited by, 30–31
Susan (case study), 33–34
systems of meaning, alterations in, 35
Szwarcberg, S., 17

T
Teicher, M., 128–29
Tenenbaum, G., 43
Tener, D., 20
terror, 88–89
thalamic dysfunction, 39–40
thoracic outlet syndrome, 51–59
thought-labels, avoiding, 158
time-limited treatment, 199
trans-generational trauma, 26–27
trauma. *See also* disclosure of abuse
childhood sexual abuse as example of, 10–12
Oliver (case study), 4–8
overview, 1–3
professional response to, 8–10
symptoms of, 3–8
trauma history, taking, 184
trauma-informed system
components of, 190–95
integrated practice, 182–84
medical training, 177–79
Olivia (case study), 187–88
overview, 175–77
personal issues for health care providers, 184–88
practice, 179–82
recognizing and reporting of abuse, 188–90
trauma quadrangle, 96–97
traumatic amnesia, 65, 82–83
trust
building of, 91–93
impact of trauma on health care relationship, 11
Oliver (case study), 4–8
as positive burden on provider, 104
safe place, building, 90, 117–18, 130–31
survivor issues with, 85
and treatment of MUS, 148–49

U
Ullman, S., 44
under-reporting of abuse, 177–78
urethral hemorrhage, 27–28
urethral pain and urgency, 76–82

V
Val (case study), 98–102
validating patient suffering, 157
van den Akker, M., 183–84
variability of telling, 17–20
ventral vagal complex, 75
veterans. *See* military trauma
vicarious traumatization, 185–86
victim-blaming, 162
victimization, 9
victim triangle, 96–97
violence
childhood sexual abuse, 10–12
Oliver (case study), 4–8
overview, 1–3
professional response to childhood trauma, 8–10
symptoms of, 3–8
Violence (Gilligan), 1–2
vomiting, 135–37
vulnerability, 88–89

W
Wagenaar, D. B., 178–79
Wain, H. J., 193

Waitzkin, H., 149–50
Walker, E., 48–49
wartime trauma. *See* military trauma
Washington trauma-informed school manual, 194–95
Wathen, C. N., 177
White, A., 18–19
Wilkinson, M., 75–76
witnessing, 200, 209
Women, Cooccurring Disorders and Violence Study (WCDVS), 190–91
written communication, 78